ACTS *of* COMPASSION

ACTS *of* COMPASSION

Bringing Love and Caring Back into Your Life

MICHAEL SPANGLE, PHD
LINDA SPANGLE, RN, MA

SunQuest
Media

Published in Denver, Colorado, by SunQuest Media.

Manufactured in the United States of America

ISBN# 979-8-9850708-1-1
e-book ISBN# 979-8-9850708-2-8

10 9 8 7 6 5 4 3

Publisher's Cataloging-In-Publication Data

Names: Spangle, Michael, author. | Spangle, Linda, author.
Title: Acts of compassion : bringing love and caring back into your life / Michael Spangle, PhD, and Linda Spangle, RN, MA.
Description: Denver, Colorado : SunQuest Media, [2022] | Includes bibliographical references.
Identifiers: ISBN 9798985070811 (paperback) | ISBN 9798985070828 (ebook)
Subjects: LCSH: Compassion. | Kindness. | Interpersonal relations.
Classification: LCC BJ1475 .S63 2022 (print) | LCC BJ1475 (ebook) | DDC 177.7--dc23

Cover Photo by Ekaterina Yakunina
Westend61

Contents

Introduction

THE WHOLE WORLD PAUSED this morning. Do you know why? Because an 8-year-old's tank was empty.

My boys were almost ready for their school day and I was preparing to leave for work when I noticed my littlest standing in the bathroom wiping his face.

I paused at the door and asked if he was okay. He looked up with tears silently dripping and shook his head. When I questioned if something happened, again he shook his head.

So I sat on the side of the tub and pulled him into my lap. I told him sometimes our heart tanks feel empty and need to be refilled.

He cried into my chest and I held tight. Then I asked if he could feel my love filling him back up. A nod, and tears stopped...

I waited a minute, then said, "Has it reached your toes yet?" He shook his head no.

"Okay then. We will take as long as you need. Work doesn't matter right now. School isn't important either. Right here, this is the most important thing today, okay? Filling you back to the top. Is that good?" He nods.

One more minute... "Is your heart full of mama's love now?" "Yeah."

I looked into his eyes and said, "I see it shining in there. You're full to the top, and you're smiling!"

You may not be 8—you may be 28, 38, 48 or whatever, but ALL of us run on empty sometimes, just like he did. His week was so busy and full and his little soul was just dry!

1

We all have to pause now and then and take a moment to refill with the good things: scripture, prayer, sunshine, worship, song, laughter, friends, hugs.

Refill your love tank when it gets empty, or you'll find emotions (tears, anger, snappy words) overflowing with no reason why.

Take a moment. Refill. It's the most important part of your day! – *Misty Starr Whittington Robertson*

IN THE SPRING OF 2021, this beautiful story was posted on Facebook by Misty Starr Whittington Robertson. Her post has been shared close to 80,000 times and has received hundreds of comments, thanking her for telling this story from her life.

We are all hungry for compassion. My goal with this book is to help you deepen your understanding of compassion and learn how to make it part of your daily life.

You will learn many ideas for showing compassion to others. But at the same time, you will discover ways to heal and renew your own spirit. And as this happens, your love tank will get filled back up.

For *Acts of Compassion* resources and free
discussion guides for churches and small groups, visit:
www.CompassionateForLife.com

CHAPTER 1

How Compassion Begins

IT WAS MY FIRST DAY of high school, and I was late.

Perhaps it was intentional, but I had started my walk to school 15 minutes later than I should have. I had been assigned to a large school that was brand new to me, and I wasn't looking forward to being there. I didn't know anyone, and I had no idea what to expect in my classes.

Once I arrived and found the correct room, I tried to slip in the door and get past the 30 students already in place. But the teacher, a big, scary-looking man with a bald head, saw me and he stopped talking. He pointed to one of the seats at the back of the full room and nodded, so I moved toward it and sat down.

After an hour of lecture, the teacher announced a short break and he headed toward my desk. I was almost shaking with fear when he stopped beside me.

But to my surprise, he didn't scold me for being late. Instead, in a calm, caring voice, he asked, "Is everything OK? Can I do anything to help?" We talked briefly and then he said, "In this class, I will be here for you. Always let me know if I can be of help in any way."

That brief gift of compassion touched my heart and totally changed my attitude. I developed a strong connection with that teacher, and he remained my friend through my four years of high school.

The compassion chair

I sometimes wonder what made that teacher's actions so important in my life. I think it's because he showed compassion at a time when I needed it most. He had no idea how alone I felt that day. But it didn't matter. He sensed that I was anxious and he reached out in a way that calmed my spirit and helped me cope.

That experience has also influenced my efforts to show compassion to others. In my work as a university professor, I began watching for students who appeared unsettled and needed someone to help them feel safe.

For many years, I had an old, faded green, overstuffed chair in my office. The chair faced away from the office door and was partially blocked by a large, fake tree. That setting helped the chair feel like a safe place for both students and staff members who came to talk.

Often the chair would be used several times during a day by people who needed to process life issues or receive a bit of help and encouragement. I also found that most of the time, the person sitting in the chair wasn't in a hurry to leave.

When someone came into the office and sat in the chair, I would simply ask, "What's going on today?" And they would talk.

I listened to stories about relationship problems, work and parenting challenges, and confessions of guilt or remorse. With each person, I attempted to show compassion as I listened to the things that were shared.

I rarely gave advice or offered solutions. Instead, I allowed my presence be the gift that each of them needed at the moment they sank into the faded chair. I suspect I helped change many lives during those green chair conversations.

Compassion reconnects

Do you have times when you feel disconnected from people in your life? It happens to everyone at times. I've heard many parents describe feeling disconnected from their kids, especially during the teen years. Even in a long-term relationship, you probably have times when you feel disconnected from your spouse or partner.

Of course, lots of things can contribute to feeling disconnected. Stress, fatigue, illness, even the weather can affect your connections with others. Feeling close again might require changing your attitude or your coping style.

But the one thing almost guaranteed to help you feel more connected is doing an act of compassion. This might be as simple as bringing home flowers or slipping your teenager some extra cash. Even the smallest demonstration of caring builds a bridge that helps you reconnect with people in your life. Try this and see what happens.

I see you

During times when you struggle with feeling hurt or upset, you can start to feel invisible. Perhaps you feel alone in the world and you might think no one even notices your pain. What you want most is for someone to "see" you and notice that you are struggling.

With my high school teacher, things changed when he saw my discomfort. First, he empathized with my feeling alone and unsafe. Then he took action by asking how I was doing and offering kind words. With that simple act of compassion, I knew that he "saw" me.

Compassion begins with you noticing someone is hurting or feeling distress. This awareness of hurt or pain prompts you

5

to feel empathy for that person, which then moves you toward doing something that addresses the discomfort.

When you display empathy and show compassion, people realize you've noticed them. Your actions demonstrate that they are not invisible and that, instead, you actually "see" them.

Seven minutes of compassion

When researchers at the California Institute of Technology studied the benefits of acts of compassion, they found an interesting pattern. They discovered seven minutes of focused compassion had a powerful effect on almost all relationships. It deepened the closeness between people and helped them let go of anger and bitterness.

The study showed that after receiving seven minutes of compassion, people noticed an increase in positive emotions such as happiness and feeling peaceful. They also reported fewer symptoms of depression, anger and sadness. Many participants described an increased sense of well-being. In other words, compassion improved people's quality of life.

Seven minutes might seem like a long time, but with planning, you will find it's not difficult to show compassion for that long. Here are a few things you can do in seven minutes:

- Write a long note or email. Include some stories about your life.
- Listen to someone without interrupting or commenting.
- Drive someone to a doctor's appointment and wait until it's finished.

One of our friends routinely goes to the home of a 98-year-old woman and sets up her medication box for the day. Then she visits for a while, makes sure this woman has her meals in place and checks to see if she needs a ride to the store or to her doctor. Our friend says that sharing those seven minutes of compassion helps both of them have a better day.

You can certainly show compassion in small ways such as holding a door for someone or calling a friend. But setting a goal of seven minutes might give you an entirely new perspective. Try the seven minutes idea and see what you notice. Create a list in a notebook or online journal of the times you showed compassion for at least seven minutes. Then evaluate the outcomes and notice how they affected your relationships.

This action can also give you a more positive outlook on your day and your life. It might make you feel more happy or peaceful, and motivate you to do it again for someone else.

Compassion changes lives

Showing compassion to others is not something new. Scientists believe that for as long as there have been human communities, compassion has been a part of life.

Psychologist Louis Cozolino says, "Humans have not thrived by survival of the fittest. Instead, they have prospered by survival of the nurtured." He believes the most successful communities and families all share the common trait of caring for those among them who are suffering.

While teaching at the University of Southern California, motivational speaker and writer Dr. Leo Buscaglia was deeply moved and saddened by a student's suicide. This led him to contemplate the ways humans become so disconnected, and he began promoting love and compassion in his classes as well as in his writing.

As the author of many books on love and caring, Buscaglia became known as "Dr. Love." He preached about love with great passion, and at his workshops, he seemed unable to stop until he had hugged everyone in sight.

He said, "Too often we underestimate the power of a touch, a smile, a kind word, a listening ear, an honest compliment, or the smallest act of caring, all of which have the potential to turn a life around."

Always remember that one simple act of compassion has the power to affect and change lives, sometimes forever.

CHAPTER 2

How Compassion Works

IN OUR SMALL TOWN IN IOWA, we live next to a row of duplex condominiums. While walking our dogs past these homes, we've met several of our neighbors, including Amber, a single mom raising a teenage daughter.

A couple summers ago, we noticed Amber had trimmed some of her trees but left the branches and leaves in a random pile next to the curb. For branches to be picked up for recycling here, they have to be cut into four-foot lengths and grouped into bundles tied with string. But week after week, the ragged pile of branches sat on the lawn next to Amber's driveway.

Finally, my wife decided to do something nice for this neighbor. So she headed to Amber's home with tree trimmers, a rake, a broom and a ball of twine. For the next couple hours, she cut the branches into short lengths and tied them in bundles.

She also raked up the leaves and debris and put them into a special bag that city staff will pick up with the trash. Finally, she swept the leftover grime off Amber's driveway and sidewalk, then gathered her tools and quietly headed back home. The next day, city workers loaded the branches and the bag of leaves into their truck and took them away.

My wife felt good about doing an act of compassion for someone, and she did not expect a thank-you or other response. In fact, the house had looked quiet the day she worked on this project, and she assumed that Amber wasn't home.

Several days later, my wife and I took our dogs for a walk and noticed Amber pulling weeds in her front yard. We stopped to say hello and chatted briefly before getting ready to continue our walk. But Amber stopped us and said, "I know what you did, and I want to say thank you."

When we asked what she meant, Amber replied, "I was inside my home watching you the whole time you were cleaning up my branches. But I was crying so hard that I couldn't come out and say thank you. No one has ever done anything that nice for me, especially people I don't even know. And I appreciated it so much." With that, she jumped up and hugged us both.

Simple acts of compassion will often bring a rainbow into people's lives and can totally change their day as well as their outlook. And many times, you won't ever know what your actions meant to those who received your compassion.

How it starts

Compassion begins with an empathetic response to the distress or suffering of another person. In some cases, the needs are obvious. But often, you simply get a sense that someone needs a little help or kindness. Then you take steps to do mindful and intentional behaviors that show you care about the wellbeing of another person.

Compassion doesn't happen in isolation. Instead, acts of compassion occur as a response to someone's need or dilemma. Here are three steps or factors involved with an act of compassion:

Step 1: NOTICE

The first step in showing compassion is noticing someone needs help. It might be an ill friend who needs transportation or a meal. Maybe an exhausted new mother needs help caring for a fussy baby. Perhaps your teen is struggling with math and is worried about failing the class.

In our busy lives, it's easy to look the other way and hope things work out for these people. On the other hand, you can notice someone's need and respond by reaching out and providing help or guidance. This means paying attention to the child who looks forlorn or helping the neighbor whose trash container fell over.

Obviously, in your normal life, you can't do this all day long. But when distress signals pop up nearby, take a look. Pay attention and notice the situation.

Sometimes you'll respond to obvious distress, hardship or suffering. Other times, it's as simple as picking up a napkin or package dropped on the floor. In many cases, you can show compassion with words of encouragement, a gentle touch or even a surprise gift.

Noticing a need can happen in an instant as you hold a door open for someone or greet a fellow church member. But other times, as in the situation with our neighbor Amber, it might take weeks or months to realize there's a need.

Often we get preoccupied with our own troubles and forget to pay attention to how other people are doing. We may think, "I'm tired. I don't have the time. I don't want to get involved. I don't know what to say or do." And we do nothing.

Of course, sometimes there are good reasons not to stop and care for another. Perhaps the situation doesn't feel safe or people don't appear open to our actions. But if we become too cautious and constantly look the other way, we can miss a lot of miracles and the joy that comes from helping others.

Compassion's power begins with truly seeing people where they are, slowing down long enough to be emotionally present and letting others know you recognize their need.

Step 2: FEEL

Compassion also requires empathy, which involves being emotionally moved by misfortune or need. Instead of just thinking about someone's problem, you bring empathy forward and actually feel something in response to the situation.

Suppose a few miles from where you live, a house catches fire. As you watch the images on the TV news, you think about how awful that must be for the family who is losing their home. You might feel sad for them and what they are going through. Right now, you are feeling sympathy. But at that point, no one is benefitting from your sadness.

But later that evening, you research the address and realize the home was close to where your kids go to school. In fact, your child is in the same class as one of the family members. As you picture that child not having school clothes or books, you consider how you would feel if your own child lost all belongings.

Your sadness builds and you sense how painful it must be for this family. In fact, you might squirm a little as you imagine the horrors of this house fire and the family's great losses. Now you are feeling empathy.

Your heart gets involved and you begin to think about how you could help them in some way. Empathy requires putting yourself in their shoes and imagining what's going on with them.

Of course, this level of emotion takes energy. If you are worn out, overwhelmed, or highly stressed, you might shut down those feelings. But even if you don't do anything right away, feeling empathy for a situation helps you stay aware of the need for compassion.

Step 3: TAKE ACTION

The natural step after feeling empathy is to take action or do something. You consider ways to help relieve the distress or suffering of others. You want people to know they are not alone and someone cares about their pain.

An act of compassion doesn't need to be a big, life changing gift. Sometimes it's simply to offer words of encouragement and support. Another time it might include a physical response where you do something that will help with the problem.

In the case of the house fire, you could donate a box of clothing and household items. Maybe you could bring the family some food or purchase a gift card for groceries. As you send or deliver your gifts, you complete the important third step—you do something.

Without that step, an act of compassion does not exist. While it's great that you notice or have feelings about someone's pain or suffering, taking action brings compassion to life.

Sympathy or empathy

Here's an important distinction. While having sympathy for someone might seem virtuous, it keeps you distant and sets you above another person's problem. On the other hand, empathy puts you on the same level and sends a critical message that says, "You are not alone."

13

Sympathy involves feeling *for* someone, but empathy becomes feeling *with* that person. With empathy, you don't judge or criticize. You simply try to understand what someone is feeling, and in that action step, empathy connects you to the person you care about.

One of my favorite authors, Dr. Brené Brown, says, "Rarely can a response make something better. What makes something better is connection."

When someone has a loss such as the death of a family member, sympathy says, "That's too bad." Empathy visits the family, brings a gift or a card, and sits with them, sometimes without speaking.

Acts of compassion don't involve trying to provide a solution or make the person feel better. Instead, you demonstrate that you are "with" that person by saying, "I will listen if you want to talk. Otherwise, I will just be here for you."

Compassion requires courage

Noticing distress or suffering doesn't happen automatically. You have to mentally slow down, pay attention and be willing to notice what's going on.

A true act of compassion doesn't require a reward or even a thank-you. Knowing someone appreciates your concern or your help might be nice. But if you are dependent on a response or a return action, you will usually be disappointed.

Acts of compassion don't have an agenda. Your goal with showing compassion is not to bring glory to yourself but to generously and openly share your gifts of concern and caring.

The reason for compassion

In our busy world, it's easy to ignore the needs of those around us. Yet compassion affects every aspect of our lives and when we do it well, it creates miracles.

As you regularly practice showing compassion, it will eventually become an attitude and a way of life. Over time, you will grasp why compassion is so important, and you will naturally identify yourself as a compassionate person. It will become part of who you are.

Build a habit of watching every day for opportunities to show compassion. Then follow the three steps:

NOTICE, FEEL, DO.

CHAPTER 3

The Power of Presence

FOR MY LUTHER SEMINARY INTERNSHIP, I worked at a church in a small town in northern Montana. The people in my church were wonderful, and they made sure my wife and I were taken care of.

In my visits with parishioners, I got to know a delightful elderly lady named Mrs. Lothian. She lived in a cute little house on the edge of town, and I visited her often. She usually made me a cup of tea and I would sip it during our visits.

But I was in my early 20s and still learning about many aspects of life. One day I received a call from Mrs. Lothian's daughter, who told me her mother was in the hospital. She said, "My mom is dying and she asked to see you."

Wow! I had never been near anyone who was dying. In fact, at that time, I had never attended a funeral. But even though I felt uneasy, I agreed to go to the hospital and visit her mom.

When I entered Mrs. Lothian's hospital room, I noticed the lights were dimmed and the white-haired lady in the bed looked small and weak. But when she saw me, she greeted me with a smile and asked me to sit in the chair beside her.

I sat down and we talked quietly for a few minutes. But I noticed she kept looking up at the far right corner of her room. Then she said, "Look, the angels are coming to get me."

I didn't know how to respond to that so I quickly stood and said, "I better get your doctor or a nurse." But she reached out and touched my arm. Then she said, "No, please stay. You are enough."

I sat down again and simply stayed with her. We talked a little and I said a prayer for God to be with her during this time. After about ten minutes, she closed her eyes and appeared to drift off to sleep.

At that point, I headed for the nurses' station and told them I thought she might need some help *now*. While I waited, the nurse headed into the room but soon came back out and told me Mrs. Lothian had died.

My heart broke and tears slipped down my cheeks! I had intended to offer a gift of compassion but it turned out that I received a greater gift from her. I will always remember her calming words with the promise, "You are enough."

It seems that instead of deep words of comfort, all she needed at that moment was my presence. And as I sat with her, she was able to relax into the arms of the angels.

Presence is a gift

Many times in life, you may not have the right words or know what to do. But just being present with someone becomes a gift.

At another time in my early ministry years, I received a panicked call from a friend who told me his 12-year-old son had been hit by a car. He asked me to come to the hospital right away. I agreed, but I couldn't help wonder what would I say at this difficult time.

When I entered the hospital room, I saw the husband and wife and three older children standing around the bed. At this point, the boy was on life support, and once again, my heart broke for this family.

I found all the medical equipment really daunting, and I had no idea what it was like to lose a child. Most of all, I didn't

17

know what to say to this hurting family. Then I remembered the words I had heard in a hospital room many years before, "Please stay, you are enough."

So I stayed. Over the next hour, we shared memories about the boy's life. We talked about the hard choices this family was facing. We spoke of God's love for their son, and I prayed with the family.

When the time came for the staff to turn off the life-support machines, we all cried together. That day, I was reminded that simply being present helps us share the suffering and tragedies of life.

What do I say?

When you become aware of someone who is suffering or in distress, you might feel totally inadequate with the idea of showing compassion. Besides that, you worry about saying the wrong thing, so you stay silent. Sometimes, you might even hesitate to show up for a visit because you aren't sure if it's appropriate.

When someone goes through a hardship such as a death, a relationship break-up or losing a job, don't worry about what to say. Instead, simply focus on being present. When possible, visit the people who had the loss or spend time with their family members and friends.

Whether you meet in person or connect in other ways, offer love and concern, not solutions. Resist the temptation to try to "make them feel better." Instead, trust that your presence will provide help and support for the journey.

Here are a few things that are always appropriate to say:

- I'm sorry for what happened.
- I'm sad for what you are going through.

- I'm here with you. I'll stay as long as you want.
- Let me know how I can be of help.

On the other hand, here are a few things it's better to not say:

- It's God's will that this happened.
- You will get over it in time.
- You can always... (have another baby, find another spouse, get another job).

Don't say "At least..."

When offering support after a loss or a life challenge, try never to start your comments with the words, "At least..." In your efforts to give comfort, you might think it will help to remind people that it could be worse. So you say, "*At least* they didn't suffer.*" Or you remind them, "*At least* your car can be replaced.*"

If those who experience the loss say "at least...," go ahead and agree with them. But don't start by saying those comments. Instead, trust that being present and saying "I care" will communicate your compassion.

You don't know how someone feels

Another statement to avoid is, "I know how you feel because I lost my... grandmother, job, cat." You don't know. If you've been through a similar loss, you know how *you* felt. But don't assume other people feel the same way you did.

To show compassion, you could say, "Even though I went through a similar loss, I can't imagine how you feel right now. I am here for you and willing to listen if that will help."

Let go of your fears about not knowing what to say. In fact, many times you won't need to say much of anything.

19

Never forget that your presence alone can become an act of compassion.

The power of "touch points"

At times, you may wonder if your actions are too insignificant to make any difference. But even the smallest acts of compassion can provide comfort and support. Every "touch point" or tiny action counts and might be the one that affects someone's life forever.

Mailing a card or writing an encouraging email or text can let people know you care about what they are going through. You don't need to make it a long message. Just tell them you are sorry, you feel sad for them or you know they are having a hard time.

When my wife's mother passed away, her friend Suzanne sent a sympathy card. In it she had written, "Losing a mother is AWFUL!" She added a couple lines about how she felt sad and how she would be happy to talk if my wife needed to.

Since then, my wife has sent out cards to many people whose mothers have died. She always starts by saying, "Losing a mother is AWFUL." Then she adds a few words of kindness and compassion.

She has found that even if women haven't been close to their mothers, there's something extra sad about a mother's death. Having someone acknowledge that brings comfort and healing.

With your children, not every event needs to be a teaching moment. Sometimes it's fine to let them work through issues by themselves. Simply watch for times when you can do a small "touch point" that shows you care about them.

Sometimes a hug or a kind word will be more effective than enforcing rules. Your kids will remember your presence more than your lessons.

Give me one minute

You don't need an hour to show compassion. Even a few seconds of kindness may be enough to help someone feel noticed or comforted. When someone has experienced a loss, simply acknowledging their sadness is a way to show compassion.

When you are really busy but you notice a person who is hurting or struggling, consider doing the *one-minute solution*. That means you give one full minute to the person in need, even if you are in the middle of a busy day.

During my ministry years, a woman named Sandy told me about her hospital stay when she'd had emergency surgery for a tubal pregnancy. Sadly, her doctor had informed her that because of other complications, she would not be able to get pregnant again.

Sandy and her husband had no other children, so this was devastating. As she struggled to deal with this news, Sandy curled up in her hospital bed and sobbed.

At one point, a nurse came into the room to adjust the IV flow and noticed Sandy was crying. The nurse asked, "Are you all right?"

Through her tears, Sandy replied, "No, I'm not." The nurse looked at her briefly, then said "OK" and left the room. At that moment, Sandy didn't need a big talk by a trained therapist. All she yearned for was one minute of compassion.

The nurse could have stood by the bedside, put her hand on Sandy's shoulder and let her know that she saw her sadness.

Perhaps she could have offered a few comments about how she was sorry for what Sandy was going through or how she cared about this huge loss.

That small demonstration of compassion would have taken only *one minute* out of her busy day. But it would have changed everything for Sandy and helped her feel not so alone in her loss.

Years ago, I heard a story about a little girl who walked to her friend's house to play. When she was late coming home, her worried mother asked what had happened and why her daughter hadn't come home sooner. The little girl said, "I'm sorry I'm late. But my friend's doll broke and I stayed to help her cry."

Never underestimate the power of your presence when people need compassion. Instead, be willing to stay and help them cry. Even a few minutes of sitting quietly with a person who is suffering or has been through a loss can bring comfort and healing.

CHAPTER 4

Compassion
Heals and Connects

IN MY EARLY YEARS as a youth pastor, I participated in a weekend conference for high school students. We had a great time with lots of good music and inspirational talks. But on the second day, I noticed a teenage girl sitting by herself on the lawn. She was curled up with her head on her knees, and I could see she was crying.

Since I was new at this, I wasn't sure what to do. But I drew on a rare bit of courage and sat down beside her. Then I gently asked, "Is everything OK?" She sat very still for a couple minutes, then said, "You don't want to know."

I replied, "Yes, I do, and I'm here for you."

Then she began to talk and spilled out her story of being sexually abused in her home by her older brother. She said she had never told anyone about this and was afraid to share it even with me.

After I listened for a while, I said I would like to help her work on this and get some resolution. Together, we made a phone call to her mother who agreed to having a family meeting that afternoon.

With my encouragement and support, the teen was able to tell her parents about the abuse and ask for help. Her brother was part of the meeting, and together, the entire family agreed to see a counselor and work on this issue.

Over the next year, this family did some amazing work and brought healing to this difficult situation. The teen became more confident and strong, and eventually went to college and completed a degree in special education.

As I reflect on this event, I believe my brief moment of compassion gave this teen hope that her life could get better. It also helped heal the relationships in this troubled family. I still hear from the student around holidays and can tell she has become an amazing wife, parent and teacher.

When people feel like giving up because of challenging situations, compassion can restore their hope for a better life. Hope increases resiliency by reminding people that they are bigger than the problems they face. It also inspires people to work on their issues instead of allowing negative events to have power over them.

Compassion doesn't discount the reality of suffering. But through words of hope, it helps people realize they are strong enough to find a way through it.

Compassion affects relationships

Along with giving hope, compassion helps improve relationships of all types. It helps bring longevity and warmth to relationships with spouses and partners. With friendships, compassion helps people manage loneliness and depression.

In families, compassion promotes a sense of security and safety in adults as well as children. Even children possess the ability to give and receive compassion. We also know that in families where compassion is freely expressed, children develop strong attachments to their parents or caregivers.

Children who don't grow up in that type of home may struggle with their capacity for empathy and compassionate behavior. Those who miss developing their compassionate heart will sometimes struggle with attachment issues even as adults.

In their efforts to discipline their children, many parents use messages that inhibit childhood compassion. When you were growing up, you probably heard at least a couple of these statements:

- Stop crying or I'll give you something to cry about.
- Grow up and act your age.
- You know that doesn't really hurt.

On the other hand, acknowledging a child's situation and giving positive messages can help promote development of compassion. Here are a few examples:

- That has to hurt! Would a hug make it feel better?
- I see you are sad. What's bothering you?
- I'm sorry you are having a hard time. Let me sit with you until you feel better.

These compassionate messages allow children to feel normal in spite of difficult circumstances. With the support of someone who cares, children learn early on how to cope with sadness or pain. They also begin to develop confidence in their ability to recover from negative feelings or events.

How we learn compassion

When one of my nephews was around three years old, he would start to wail and cry whenever he was put into his car seat. One day, his mother demonstrated how his teddy bear was able to calm itself by putting its paws together and thinking quiet thoughts.

They practiced this a couple times, and my nephew loved how this worked. After that, whenever she put my nephew into his car seat, she would say, "Now, just like your teddy bear, put your little hands together and calm yourself."

As he did that, he tried to think quiet thoughts and he was able to stop himself from crying. That compassionate approach helped my nephew learn he could manage his discomfort and let go of his sad feelings.

Most of us can recall special moments when our parents did something nice for us. You might remember a special childhood birthday party or the day you got the new shoes you really wanted. These moments leave a lasting memory that helps us understand and appreciate compassion.

For many of my younger years, my mom made a big deal out of Easter morning. I would always wake up to an elaborate Easter basket on the end of my bed. It had a chocolate rabbit, some candy eggs and even a couple of little gifts. I can still recall how happy I felt when I reached for that Easter basket.

My mother's small act of compassion gave me a wonderful memory that I cherish to this day. In an often troubled childhood, that simple gift also gave me hope that things would get better.

Compassion strengthens relationships

Our inner spirits yearn for friends who stand by us, empathize with our pain and reach out a helping hand. I love music and have found that it often brings me healing and comfort as well as enjoyment.

Many of my favorite songs talk about how compassion builds strong friendships. I love the messages in the Simon and Garfunkel song *Bridge over Troubled Water* and Mariah Carey's *Anytime You Need a Friend*.

The lyrics in these songs remind us that a good friend will be there for us, dry our tears, and never walk away when we need help or support.

Our friendships in life make up an integral part of our social wellbeing, but compassion is what keeps them strong. We see it when friends pause from the burdens of their life to hear about our issues. We also experience it when a friend listens without judgment and calms us with reassuring words.

During the challenging times of life, we value a friend who spends time with us, acknowledges our pain and listens without offering solutions. Think about times when a friend has gone extra steps to be a help to you.

A compassionate friend will often do some of these things:

- Change plans in order to be there for us during a time of need.
- Listen to us and acknowledge our disappointment, sadness, or anxiety.
- Say, "That would hurt me too!" or "I'm sorry that happened to you."

In my classes and groups, I've done surveys to find out what people believe is the most important quality for developing strong relationships. Their answers would usually include things such as someone I can trust, someone who supports me or someone who listens.

What surprised me was that the quality that nearly always showed up on the list was a friend displaying warmth. This included things such as giving a kind, valuing smile or looking directly into someone's eyes to show caring. Sometimes it was a handshake or a hug that gave the message, "I'm glad to see you."

In friendships as well as marriages, compassion helps deepen the quality and strength of the relationship. In a study published in the journal *Emotion*, the authors found that compassion is the most important quality of a successful long-term relationship. The study listed helpful behaviors such as offering words of encouragement and support during a difficult time or understanding the stress of a traumatic event.

Long-term effects of compassion

I was eight years old when my parents divorced. It was a sad time for a little boy who now didn't have his father to greet him when he woke up in the morning or kiss him before bed at night.

He had just taught me to ride my bike without the training wheels. He had also bought me a used baseball glove, and he was helping me learn to play catch. I was hoping he'd teach me to use the bat as well. But now he was gone.

When Christmas season came that year, I wanted to give my father something special but didn't have much money. From my piggy bank, I was able to come up with $2. But I kept wondering what kind of gift I could buy with that small amount.

I don't recall the name of the store, but I remember the purchase. I found a little figurine with a boy and father that met my budget. I bought it, wrapped it in festive paper and gave it to my father for Christmas.

I never thought much about that figurine until my dad died, 60 years later. While going through his belongings, I discovered that figurine on a bookshelf above his work desk. As a young boy, I gave him that gift out of my deepest compassion, and I was amazed to see that he had treasured it all his life.

Sometimes we underestimate the power of compassion. But we know that it builds deeper relationships and enables people to stand together against life challenges such as health problems, job loss and family struggles. Often your most important words might be, "Other people have gotten through this, and so can you." Or you can say, "I may not get everything right, but I will be here and help you with this."

These messages build a sense of hope that the relationship can remain strong. It reminds your loved one, "I share your hurt and you can lean on me until it's over."

With struggling relationships, compassionate acts can bring healing and comfort. These might be as small as tucking a note into a briefcase or sending an email or text saying, "I miss you today." Sometimes it might involve planning a special night out or taking over a hard task that gives relief to another's burdens.

Compassion shows grace

Over the years, I have been "sort of" a golfer. Many days at the golf course, I hit the ball everywhere but where I want it to go. Even though I have years of learning and practice, I'm still embarrassed when I hit the ball into a lake or into the trees.

My favorite golf partners are people who also have bad days and show me some grace. When I have a terrible shot, they usually say, "Oh, that's got to hurt. We'll call that a mulligan." I'm always relived because that word means I get the shot over. Because I feel accepted and encouraged, I hit the ball again and hope that some day I will improve.

Grace in relationships works the same way. Perhaps you feel anxious about making a special dinner, doing a home project or trying to explain something that's important to you.

But a compassionate partner or friend accepts us with grace and encourages us to keep at it. Even when we feel inadequate, compassion helps us tackle the challenge.

In all types of relationships, the expression of grace becomes a core element of compassionate behavior. Showing grace helps us know that someone understands us and accepts us in spite of our weakness. A compassionate friend affirms our worth by allowing our failures and encouraging us to keep working on our challenges.

Emotional availability

How often do you find that a friend or partner seems constantly preoccupied with things other than you? After a while, you realize the person is not available for you emotionally, and you start pulling away from the relationship.

You probably recognize when people are doing avoidance behaviors. They look away a lot, they glance at their phone or their watch, or they seem to have something more important to do. They don't take the time to invest in the friendship or relationship.

In a secure relationship, you feel confident that when you need it the most, someone will be there for you. Being emotionally available requires shutting off distractions and making someone's needs the most important thing of the moment. When you are spending time with someone, make every effort to silence your cell phone and ignore texts and notices. Every time you glance at your phone, you disconnect emotionally from the person you are with.

Showing gratitude

Whether you are expressing or receiving compassion, showing gratitude significantly improves your relationships. All of us want to feel appreciated and valued, and showing gratitude gives us a way to do this.

A few years ago, one of my staff members went through an especially demanding time with her job. In my efforts to care about this employee, I gave her extra time to work on her projects and tried to support and encourage her whenever I could. Eventually, her work demands slowed down and she seemed fine again.

Several months later, she sent me a lovely card with a handwritten note that said, "Thank you so much for all your help and support through my work situation. I know you understood the events that affected me because you've been there. I appreciate how you supported me while I was going through that tough time."

Her simple note made my day! I hadn't realized that I'd helped her that much, and her words made me feel valued and appreciated.

Even showing gratitude for someone's presence helps strengthen relationships. Over the many years of our marriage, my wife and I will often say to each other, "I'm glad you're in my life."

CHAPTER 5

Compassion Helps Both People

SHOWING COMPASSION typically seems like a one-sided event. You see a need, feel empathy, and take action. While you might not always know whether your compassion was helpful, many times you'll be rewarded with a smile or a thank-you. Then you move on and go back to your regular life.

But what happened inside your own heart and spirit? Did you feel a bit happier or more content after you cared about someone? Perhaps you noticed your own steps picked up a little or you smiled as you walked away.

The Center for Compassion and Altruism at Stanford University has published many studies on the outcomes of showing compassion. Their research shows that compassionate acts benefit people who give them as well as those who receive them.

When we broaden our perspective beyond ourselves, we quietly improve our own lives. As we offer compassion to another, studies show there is a reduction in activity of the parasympathetic nervous system. This decreases blood pressure and the level of inflammatory proteins linked to heart disease. In other words, showing compassion can improve our health and even strengthen our immune system.

By nature, our minds tend to focus on what is negative, but compassion draws us into a realm of seeing the good around us. Through our compassionate acts, we give others hope at the same time we instill a greater hope in ourselves. So even our small acts of kindness and support make a significant contribution to our own good health.

Windsailing and compassion

Many years ago, my father made a rare visit to Colorado, and we both worked on being kind and feeling closer to each other. At one point, he offered to teach me windsailing, which was his favorite sport where he lived in California.

On a nice windy day, we headed out to a large lake. First he gave me a basic lesson on how to balance on what looks like a surfboard. Then he showed me how to grip the heavy mast which held the sail.

I carefully got into the water and climbed on the board. As I stood up and grabbed on to the mast, the wind caught the sail and off I went out on the lake. However, I wasn't strong enough to hold the mast in a way that allowed me to shift directions, so I could make only left turns.

As I sailed off down the lake, I quickly realized I was getting far away from the shore, and I couldn't figure out how to turn around. Finally I managed to maneuver the board closer to the shore, where I got down and paddled toward the sandy beach.

I was exhausted and had no idea how I was going to get back to where we had started. It seemed that I had to either carry the heavy board along the shore for an hour or push myself back out onto the lake.

At that moment, I looked up and saw my father walking along the shore to help me, and I realized he had been watching me the entire time. My eyes filled with tears as I recognized my father's compassion, and that event brought us much closer in the remaining years before his death.

Sometimes, compassion helps both people by demonstrating the importance of someone being there for us when we need it. That experience with my father showed me the power of compassion in relationships, even ones that are distant. And it reminded me to work harder at showing compassion to others, including people I'm not close to in my life.

Compassion at work

In work settings, creating and sustaining relationships often plays a critical role in accomplishing the goals of a job. Organizational behavior research shows that demonstrating concern for co-workers can improve productivity and cooperation.

It appears that people feel better about their jobs when they believe others are supportive during times of high stress and demands. We also know that employee retention and job satisfaction are higher in organizations that foster compassion.

In their company mission statement, the UnitedHealth group includes the goal of demonstrating compassion to others. Here's how they express its importance:

*We try to walk in the shoes of the people we serve
and the people we work with across the health care
community. Our job is to listen with empathy and
then respond appropriately and quickly with service
and advocacy for each individual, each group or
community, and for society as a whole.*

Appreciation of employees

A few years ago, I was asked to help a hospital catheterization lab that was struggling with high tension and conflict between the doctors, nurses and technicians. Much of their work involved inserting tubes into hearts to visualize the arteries and treat abnormalities. Because the staff worked so closely together, these tasks required a lot of cooperation between the team members.

The technicians and nurses described being on their feet for long periods of time, doing critical procedures and dealing with the constant noise from the lab machines.

Many of them sounded discouraged and generally unhappy. When I asked what they needed most, I expected to hear they needed more breaks or wanted additional time off. But instead, they all agreed, "We just want to be appreciated for the work we do. We don't think doctors understand the important contribution we make."

These staff members wanted to receive empathy and gratitude from the cardiac doctors for the extra work involved in this lab. Then they explained, "The best symbol of how little the doctors value us is their annual Christmas gift which is a barrel of stale popcorn."

What this team really wanted was to be appreciated and have this shown in ways that involved more than popcorn. In my discussion with the physicians, we realized that lack of showing compassion was at the center of this relationship breakdown. Fortunately, the doctors were open to this insight, and they agreed to show more caring and appreciation for the work of the staff members.

Medical settings present a lot of challenges with trying to show compassion while delivering high-level patient care. But research has found that when nurses demonstrate compassion in their work, it reduces patient loneliness, eases anxiety and builds trust in the medical team.

In fact, research shows that compassionate relationships can result in measurable differences in health care outcomes. In 2018, one medical study found that patients who received just 40 seconds of compassion a day expressed less fear and anxiety. Another study found that heart patients who received compassionate care were less likely to die over the next year.

Compassion relieves loneliness

During my work as a Navy Chaplain, I spent a few weeks at a hospital on the West Coast. One morning, a doctor asked if I could help with an older man who was in serious condition. This patient was depressed and had refused to take his heart medication. He wouldn't talk to anyone and appeared to have lost hope of getting better.

I went to see the man and found him sitting alone in the middle of his room with his head down. I noticed there were no get well cards, no flowers, and no TV or music playing. I pulled a chair up in front of him and when I called him by name, he lifted his head. But for a while, he wouldn't speak or respond to me.

Finally, I asked him where he was from, and he quietly said, "Montana." I told him that I had lived in Montana for a year, and I asked what he did there before he retired. He answered, "I worked on the railroad."

For the next fifteen minutes, we talked about the beauty of Montana and his work for many years on the railroad. When I asked about his family, he explained they were all in Montana and too far away to visit him in the hospital. I could see how much he missed the land, his family and his life back home.

I know he felt my compassion for his being so far away from his family and the home he loved. When I asked if he wanted to eventually go home, he said, "Oh, yes, I'd love to. But I've given up hope of doing that."

Realistically, I knew he might not be able to get back home, but I said, "Well, let's try again. You belong *there*, not *here*. During my weeks of duty here, I will come and visit with you every day until you can go back home."

Then I added, "Would you be willing to let the nurses help you with your medicine?" He nodded and thanked me for being his friend.

I realized this man wanted someone to understand his loneliness and sadness, but not give him orders about what to do. He wanted someone who would listen to his story and value what was important to him.

My act of compassion in talking with this man gave him some hope that his health might improve enough that he could go back home. But that experience also provided me with some wonderful learning and inspiration about how to help others who have lost hope. In this situation, both of us benefitted from my compassion.

Compassion with pets

My wife and I have been parents to quite a few dogs over the years. We are often amazed at how these animals receive as well as give compassion. We try to give them a lot of caring and attention, and in return, they wag their tails and show us love.

When one of us has been ill, our dogs seem to sense our pain and will sit quietly next to us as we recover. I remember how one of my favorite cocker spaniels would lie in a chair next to me with her head on my chest. In that simple action, she gave me amazing comfort.

One friend described how when she had a migraine or was in pain, her cat would jump on the bed and curl around her.

I've also seen amazing outcomes with comfort dogs who have been trained to visit people in hospitals and nursing homes. Even when patients are very ill, their faces light up when a compassionate dog sits at their side or puts its head on their laps.

Compassion changes us

In my years as a minister, I took many youth groups on compassion trips to help build or repair homes. We painted, cleaned, sorted and carried trash for elderly, ill and disabled individuals who weren't able to do these things on their own.

I was always amazed at the transformation I saw in the teenagers during these mission trips. Often they would talk about how this work revived their own spirits and gave them a better outlook on life.

Scott Pious, a professor at Wesleyan University, ends his psychology courses with a "Day of Compassion." He asks students to live as compassionately as they can for 24 hours, then write about their experiences. The students create stories that tell of improved family relationships, getting to know neighbors, and being inspired to continue living as compassionate individuals.

As a university professor, I've heard a lot of graduation speeches. Most of them were dull and forgotten by the time the ceremony was over. But one year, I heard a commencement speech that stuck with me long term.

Regis University President Father Mike Sheeran said, "Your final test from this university is not how well you did on the exams and written papers for your courses. It's how you choose to live your life and the lives you influence."

He concluded his talk by challenging the students to demonstrate compassion for all those the world may have forgotten and strive to be remembered as someone who cared.

Mother Teresa

Nun and missionary Mother Teresa, known in the Catholic church as Saint Teresa of Calcutta, devoted her life to caring for the sick and poor. As one of the greatest humanitarians of the 20th century, Mother Teresa had an unwavering commitment to aiding those most in need.

During her lifetime, she showed compassion toward thousands of people, and she challenges us to continue her work forever. She left us with these words:

Let no one ever come to you without leaving better and happier. Be a living expression of God's kindness— kindness in your face, kindness in your eyes, kindness in your smile. – Mother Teresa

CHAPTER 6

Stories Behind the People

WE KNOW SOMEONE WELL, or at least, we think we do. Then one day, we learn about a recent tragedy, sadness or loss in that person's life. We are shocked! We had no idea what they were going through, and we just assumed they were fine.

Behind every person is a story. Whether it's your closest friends, family members or people you work with, everyone's life contains lots of stories. When we stop and listen, we might hear people describe joy and happiness. But we also might hear about disappointment, sadness and heartbreak.

Of course, we don't need to know someone's whole life story in order to show compassion. But it's easy to miss the important details and think we have someone all figured out. Unfortunately, a lot of the time we are wrong.

It's not how it looks

When I was teaching an evening graduate class, one student showed up a half hour late for the first two weeks of class. I wanted to be kind so I didn't say anything to her about it. I thought perhaps she'd gotten stuck in traffic or had problems at her work. But then I noticed she didn't seem to know any of the other students, and she also left class a half hour early.

The third week, she came in late again and didn't bring the week's assignment. I assumed she wasn't a good student or she wasn't committed to her work in this class. So I decided it was time to have a hard conversation.

40

During the break, I went over to her and said, "You seem to be struggling a bit with this class. Is everything okay? Can I be of help?"

She answered, "I live in a homeless shelter at night and have to ride the bus to get here. It only comes at inconvenient times, so that's why I'm late. Then I have to leave class early to get on the bus to go home. And this week, I couldn't get time on the community library computer so I couldn't finish tonight's assignment."

Then she shared that she was a victim of abuse by her husband. She was basically homeless and had moved into the shelter in order be safe. Now I felt embarrassed by my quick judgments about her and decided it was time to show some compassion. I told her I understood and would look for ways to help make this class work for her.

With her permission, I told the class a little of the student's story and her current struggles. Then I watched my small caring actions mushroom into class compassion. By the end of that evening, the other students had grouped together to provide some help for this woman. They agreed to share their evening snacks, pick her up for class and take her home afterward.

Two years later, I got teary-eyed as I watched that student receive her college degree. She now had a good job and lived in an apartment. Our class became a part of helping her achieve her dream. It demonstrated how compassion can help repair people's lives and give them a second chance.

Learn the story

So many times in life, I have made assumptions or judgments about people, then learned these were completely wrong. Now I often remind myself that behind every painful or uncomfortable situation, there's a story. I may not always be able to find out the details or learn the background of those I try to help. But taking time to learn more about others feels like an essential part of my efforts to show compassion.

Some years ago, I had an administrative assistant whose work had gone downhill. Where she had previously completed tasks on time and done good quality work, now she kept getting behind and not following through on work assignments. Some days she came to work late without giving an explanation.

As time went on, I became irritated and wondered if I needed to confront her about these work issues. One day, after I'd chided her about the way I wanted something done, I noticed she was trying to avoid crying.

At first, I didn't want to deal with her problems, and my perception was that she didn't want to work for me any more. But finally, I softened and asked her what was wrong. She quietly told me that while she was at work, her daughter was skipping school and meeting friends at the mall. She was a single mom and didn't have anyone else to help her deal with her daughter.

Again, I realized how easy it is to judge people when you don't know their story. I quickly shifted my approach and let her know I was sorry for her struggle and I cared about her and her daughter. Then we arranged for her to take some extra time off and have more flexibility in her hours until things improved.

A side benefit was that my relationship with that worker became a lot stronger once I noticed her suffering. And soon she went back to showing the wonderful work skills that made her a valuable employee.

It's not what you think

How many times do you see people who seem to be upset or struggling and you mentally assign them quick labels? Then as you spend time with them, you learn there's a different story. Sometimes we feel so sure we understand a person or situation, and we keep acting on our belief or opinion. But later we discover we were completely wrong about what was going on. When this happens to me, I feel embarrassed and frustrated that I didn't look beyond the obvious and learn more about someone.

Perhaps the grouchy person was in pain and the mean one was lonely. The boring person might be a retired engineer who holds patents on several amazing inventions. Maybe the bad parent has a newborn baby and hasn't slept much for weeks.

In my work as a chaplain, I saw many examples of inaccurate assumptions. At a large hospital in Denver, Colorado, an elderly female patient named Mary was ready to go home. But the nursing staff couldn't find the woman's clothes. They searched the room and the small closet, but the clothes bag had disappeared.

The staff gave Mary a set of hospital scrubs for her trip home and assured her they would check with the laundry department to try to find her missing clothes. Mary wasn't very happy with this approach, but since she didn't have much choice, she put on the scrubs and got into her friend's car to return home.

Once she got there, she waited for a phone call that would let her know when she could pick up her own clothes. But there was no call. A couple of days went by without any news, so Mary called the hospital to check if they had found the bag of clothes. No one seemed to have any information about this, and they told her to call back in a few days.

For several weeks, Mary kept calling and never got an answer about her missing clothes. Finally she'd had enough! She called the local newspaper and told them about her problem and how angry she was with the customer service at this hospital. Instead of putting an article in the newspaper, one of the editors called the hospital to see why it hadn't helped this woman.

After talking to people at several departments, the editor reached a nurse's aide who remembered Mary and her long stay at the hospital. The aide volunteered to try to fix this situation. When she found out that Mary lived close to her, she set up a time for a visit. When the aide arrived, Mary invited her in but immediately started to cry. As the aide comforted Mary, she asked more about what had been in the clothes bag.

Through her tears, Mary explained she didn't care about the clothes. But that bag also contained a necklace that was the last gift from her husband who had recently died. Her anger wasn't about the missing clothes. Instead, she was going through grief about losing her husband of many years.

The nurse's aide sat with her for a long time and listened to her describe her loneliness and the challenges of not having her husband to help her. Finally, Mary said she felt better, and she thanked the aide for her compassion. She also told the aide she just wanted someone to care about her, and now she was ready to let go of her anger at the hospital and move on in her healing.

In your own life, I encourage you to look beyond the obvious answer to someone's struggle. Instead, listen longer and see what else you can learn. Ask questions and get more details about someone's anger or frustration. There's a good chance you will discover the real story is far different from what you think.

Where is the pain?

As a hospital chaplain, I was often asked to help with "problem patients." According to the medical staff, many of these patients were uncooperative, refused treatments or acted rude and grouchy all the time. During my visits, I couldn't always solve the issues or improve the relationships. But I always tried to learn more about each of the patients and get a glimpse of what was behind their struggles.

The request that challenged me the most came from the staff at a large hospital in Maryland. They had a new patient who was sitting in the middle of a busy hallway with a blanket over her head. She would not respond to anyone and refused to be taken back to her hospital room. I had never worked with this type of patient and I didn't have a clue about how to help her.

When I got to the hospital floor, I saw her right away—sitting in a wheelchair with her head covered by a white blanket. Unsure of how to talk with her, I pulled a chair out from one of the nearby rooms, sat down in front of her and waited.

After a few minutes of quiet, I told her I was a chaplain and asked if I could visit with her. She grumbled something in a faint voice. So I started talking about simple things such as the weather and that it was a nice hospital, and she made small comments back.

Finally I said, "You know, we could have a much better conversation if you could remove that blanket you're wearing." She answered, "You don't want to see me." I assured her that I did. Then she slowly pulled the blanket back just a little and I could see that the skin on her face was diseased and peeling off.

I kept sitting with her and gradually she started to talk about her illness. I simply acknowledged her painful life and asked how I could help her get through this. Then she told me her family lived out of state and wouldn't arrive for another week. She said, "I'm all alone, and I don't know what to do."

At this point, I told her I wanted to help, but we could probably visit easier where it was quiet. She nodded and let me wheel her into her hospital room. As we continued to talk, she slowly began to take off the blanket. I could see she was terrified of the medical treatments and missed the help and support of her family. So I told her I would come to visit her every afternoon until her family arrived. We got to know each other and shared a lot of our life stories.

One week later, when I arrived for my visit, I found her in a meeting room, surrounded by her loving family. Her medical treatments had been working and she looked a lot better than when I had first met her. She proudly introduced me to her family members as the chaplain who had made her feel like living again.

Many times in life we meet people who are dealing with horrific medical or emotional problems. In most cases, we can't fix their situation or bring healing to their bodies. But when we look past their issues, we begin to see the real person behind the story. And our compassion might be the tiny spark that gives someone encouragement and hope for recovery.

Let go of judgments and assumptions

Every once in a while, I will quickly form an opinion about what's going on with someone. If I see some kind of odd behavior, I assume it must be because the person is old, poor, grouchy or sick.

During early December one year, I went to my favorite hobby store. While I was shopping, I noticed an elderly, frail-looking woman enter the store and begin putting lots of games and toys into a shopping cart.

I couldn't imagine who she was buying gifts for because she got duplicates of several items. But I also wondered how she was going to take all her gifts home because she didn't appear to have a car.

The woman ended up being in the checkout line in front of me, so I had to patiently wait while the store clerk rang up her purchases. He asked if she wanted everything put into bags, and she answered, "No, just put them back into the cart after you scan them." When the clerk gave her the total, she pulled out about $200 of cash and paid for the items.

Then I watched in amazement as she pushed the cart over to a large box labeled "Toys for Tots" where we could donate things for people in need. One by one, she took each of the games and toys out of her cart and put them into the large box. Then she left the store and walked slowly across the parking lot again.

As I paid for my supplies, I asked the store clerk about the woman. He said, "She comes here every year about this time and buys a lot of things for kids of every age. Then she puts them all into the Toys for Tots box. She is an amazing person and we love her."

Remember the story

When you see people who don't match your ideal culture, body size or personality style, stop your negative thoughts. Instead remember that you don't know the details of their lives. You can't see their hidden wounds caused by fears, loss or grief.

Remind yourself that all people have a story and that's what makes them unique. You don't need to fix them or even hear their story. Instead, strive to show compassion, and trust that your action has the ability to heal, comfort and encourage them, no matter what's in their story.

For many years, I had a small sign on my work desk that said, "Listen longer." It reminded me to let people tell their stories or problems without forming assumptions about them or what they needed.

Many times, I realized my first impressions about their situations were completely wrong. If I hadn't allowed them to talk longer, I would have missed the most important parts of their stories.

When you meet people who seem to be struggling in life, be patient and listen to them longer. Learning the stories behind these people will help you become more compassionate and caring toward them.

CHAPTER 7

Compassion and the Brain

ONE OF MY LONGTIME FRIENDS regularly asks me how I'm doing. I typically give a quick response of "I'm fine" even when I'm not. But usually my friend sees through me and follows her initial question by saying, "No, I want to know how you are *really* doing." Then she patiently listens as I share the details of my life.

Why does this friend listen better than most people who ask me the same question? The answer lies in the way her brain focuses its attention on others. Like a laser, she has the ability to zero in on my emotional pain and turn that attention into empathy.

When one of my favorite dogs died last year, I was devastated. I loved my dog so much, and losing her made me feel terribly sad. One morning soon after her death, I was sitting at a coffee shop when someone approached my table. I looked up and recognized one of the customers who came there often.

He stood for a moment, then said, "Are you OK? You look pretty down today." I told him about my dog and how hard it was to deal with her dying. He nodded and said, "Been through that, and it's really hard. Eventually it will be OK again." Then he gently patted my shoulder before heading out the door.

I was grateful for his compassion, but I was also amazed that he had noticed my sadness. What caused him to see that I was having a hard day? In the same way my longtime friend knew when I wasn't "fine," some people have an exceptional ability to recognize cues that things aren't quite right.

Compassion starts in your brain

The study of neuroscience helps us understand how compassion works and why it is so important in building successful relationships. Research in this field has shown that our brain has the ability to realize when things are not as they should be.

You might notice someone's slouching shoulders or hollow voice tone. When you look into a person's eyes, you might see sadness, fatigue or frustration. Recognizing these cues prompts the thought sequence and feelings of empathy that lead toward an act of compassion.

Unfortunately, it's easy to miss these signals. Our busy lives will often distract us from noticing other people's distress. Perhaps you are answering phone texts and you miss clues about a friend's loneliness or unhappiness.

Maybe you are exhausted after work and don't realize it's been awhile since you've had any deep conversations with family members. Or worry about your job or finances prevents you from seeing your upset child waiting at the door of your home office.

Recently a friend described a sad moment with his seven-year-old daughter. After asking him several times to talk with her, his daughter said, "I wish you would listen to me like you do the people you work with." He suddenly realized he was putting everything else in life ahead of his daughter's needs.

Short attention span

The neural processes in your brain work together to direct and hold your attention. But when you get overwhelmed or busy, your attention weakens.

You forget where you put your keys, you can't find your eyeglasses, or you have no idea why you went into a room. These concerns don't usually mean you're forgetful. Instead, your brain stopped paying attention and let things slip through the cracks.

Lack of attention also affects your ability to show compassion. You stop noticing people's clues of worry, fear, sadness or anxiety. Soon, opportunities go by and you realize later that you didn't show compassion when someone needed it.

To strengthen your brain's attention circuits, you need to manage distractions and focus more on the person in front of you. You also need to practice mindfulness and awareness of your surroundings. To do this, you may need to slow down and live in the present instead of waiting for a time when you aren't so busy.

Often your environment can distract you and cause you to miss subtle clues. In your home, people may have to compete with a football game or a sitcom on television. Cell phones and social media have complicated things even more.

Mary told me about joining a friend for lunch at a nice restaurant. In the middle of their visit, the friend got a text and immediately pulled out her phone to read it. She then spent the next few minutes on her phone, responding back and forth.

Finally, Mary asked, "Is there something important going on?" Her friend apologized for the interruption but explained she was confirming a lunch plan with a different friend. Mary said, "It felt like being on a date with someone and in the middle of the evening, having that person set up a date with someone else."

Practicing mindfulness

Training yourself to pay attention involves the practice of mindfulness, which focuses on moment-to-moment awareness. If you have children, you certainly know the challenges of when they are young. In an instant, a toddler can get into the cupboards, eat soap or use a permanent marker on the walls. Most parents develop a "kid radar" that stays on alert whenever their children are in the room. Somehow, they develop a strong ability to stay aware, even when there are lots of distractions and other activities.

You can develop this same skill with adults by paying more attention to details. When you get ready to leave for work, what do you notice? Does anyone look upset or stressed? Are people rushing because they're late? Do your preschool children appear happy and content or are they crying about their spilled cereal?

Practicing mindfulness helps you slow down and pause before you head out the door. By quickly monitoring your surroundings and picking up details, you will improve your awareness. And that's the step that will help you catch the times when someone needs a bit of compassion or love.

Is the danger real?

The *amygdala* area of your brain has one job. It's supposed to alert you to danger. At times, this is critical because the danger is real. If you smell smoke or a car cuts in front of you on the highway, you need to recognize the danger and take action.

Your amygdala also evaluates the people in your life. It if senses a threat, real or imagined, it can cause you to have fear or distrust. It can also prompt you to avoid people or misinterpret what they say. Your amygdala is designed to protect you, but when it fires at the wrong times, it can cause you to stay on edge.

Sometimes, after a scary event is past, your brain loses track and forgets to turn the amygdala back off. In some cases, people don't realize they are still on high alert and they live with chronic stress. Other times, the amygdala might suspect problems with a spouse or child when things are fine. These danger signals can begin to challenge people's mental health and harm relationships.

For responders such as police or firefighters, it can be challenging to let go of the fear of danger. When I worked with police personnel, I learned how hard it was for them to maintain marriage and family relationships. Because their days were filled with stress and high-alert status, it was difficult to come home, slow down, and pay attention to family members.

With war veterans, the memory of a danger threat can cause long-term struggles with post-traumatic stress disorder (PTSD) or depression. In this case, the brain continues to send threat signals, even years after the dangerous events are over. These people have to consciously train themselves to let go of fears and trust they are safe.

For some professions, creating a buffer between work and home helps force the brain to let go of stress. When a therapist friend got home from work, she would immediately go up to her bedroom and change her clothes. She taught herself to shake off the stress and angst from her day when she put her work clothes in the laundry basket.

Another professional trained his family members to give him ten minutes of alone time when he entered the house before hitting him with demands and reports about the day.

This simple routine helped his brain let go of stressful work events and prepared him to be patient and kind with his family.

The answer is green

Sometimes your amygdala gets overactive and refuses to calm down. When you feel anxious or upset, your mind starts going in all directions, and those feelings begin to increase and get worse.

Research shows that you can stop those emotions from taking over by doing something that helps you feel emotionally grounded. Here is the fastest and simplest way to do this:

Look for something *green*. Whether you're outdoors, in an office or staring at your kid's messy room, find something green to focus on. It might be a tree or plant, a book or something in a picture on a wall.

Keep focusing on what you found for a minute or so. Then look for something else that's green and focus on that. Because green is a calming and nurturing color, your brain slows down and helps you feel grounded again.

Doing this exercise won't fix the issues you are dealing with, but it buys you some time to think about your next move instead of blowing up or yelling at someone.

Where empathy begins

When you notice someone struggling and you suddenly feel empathy for that person, you have triggered the *insula* region of your brain. Neuroscience believes the insula is responsible for self-awareness, taste and perception. It also promotes understanding, caring and confidence in relationships.

Similar to the brain regions associated with attention, the insula can also be trained. Improving your ability to show empathy starts with becoming more aware of how you are responding. You can start by listening longer to what people are saying and monitoring your reactions to their words. Once you understand more about their issues, you can show them warmth and caring.

What empathy does *not* do is provide solutions. Many times in my marriage, my wife will start talking about some issue in her friendships or her work, and I quickly tell her how to fix the problem. For some reason, she doesn't seem to appreciate my help. Instead, it usually makes her mad. Finally after one of our rather poor conversations, my wife said, "I don't need you to fix this. In fact, I don't even want your insights. I just want you to listen and nod your head a lot."

We started calling this the "poor baby" response, and we both use it often. When one of us starts ranting about some issue in our day, the other one quietly says, "Poor baby." That simple phrase helps us listen and understand but not attempt to give any solutions or answers.

To become good at empathy, you have to learn how to show concern and caring without letting people's problems devastate you. Instead of immediately giving out solutions or answers, think "poor baby" and let them talk.

In my counseling work, I've had to remind myself that I'm not a repairman. My job is to listen, show empathy and guide people toward making changes in their lives. The motto that helps me the most is, "It's not your job to fix them; it's your job to love them!"

Improving empathy

As you know, empathy is the second step in acts of compassion. It also might be the most essential tool for establishing connections with people. We know the neural circuitry associated with empathy is able to learn and change. By focusing on specific details, you can teach this area of your brain to do a better job.

Here are some simple ways to improve your ability to show empathy:

- Listen longer, without interrupting.
- Seek to understand rather than provide solutions.
- Manage distractions, such as TV or texting, that can cause you to lose focus.
- Cultivate a sense of curiosity about what's going on for someone.
- Imagine what it must be like to have the problems you are hearing about.

The calm-down nerve

When you get stressed or upset, the *vagus* nerve in your brain quickly gets involved. Depending on the context or situation, this nerve strives to help regulate internal functions such as heart rate, breathing and digestion.

If you feel stressed or angry, the vagus nerve can help you lower your voice, speak softly, and approach other people in a safe and supportive manner. Calming yourself improves your ability to notice suffering, feel empathy and care for needs.

Medical personnel such as nurses and first responders train themselves to draw on this nerve during a crisis or emergency. This helps them remain calm and professional even as they deal with the most challenging situations.

To stimulate the healthy functions of the vagus nerve, practice slow, deep breathing. You can consciously slow your breathing by counting to yourself as you inhale and exhale. To deepen your breathing, attempt to exhale longer than you inhale.

For another calming exercise, take seven slow, deep breaths, but make each one slower and deeper than the one before. Most people lose track of the number of breaths before they reach number seven.

Your face looks unhappy

Another brain system connected to empathy involves the *mirror neurons*. This area enables us to read messages we see in someone's voice tone, eyes, facial expressions and body movement.

The mirror neurons enable us to imagine what life must be like for others. When someone hits a thumb with a hammer, our mirror neurons identify with the experience and cause us to wince as though we were in pain. When someone tells us about going through a medical procedure, we may say, "Oh, that's got to hurt."

People with underdeveloped mirror neurons may struggle with important relationships. They might lack the skill to see clues that communicate emotions in others. They'll probably miss nonverbal messages that indicate frustration, disappointment or fatigue.

At times all of us will have a hard time reading other people's emotions. Once we become aware of this, we can explore or clarify what someone is communicating. For example, you might say, "What I hear you saying is...." Or you might ask, "Did I get that right? Is this how you feel?" Even guessing how someone might feel can be helpful. At worst, the person will correct you and help you understand the problem.

Taking difficult action steps

Scholars who study brain behavior have found that people naturally tend to have a negative bias toward the world. We notice bad things more than good ones. For example, although you receive many positive comments about your work project, your brain drifts toward the one negative comment you heard. This negative bias can make you believe that you did a poor job in spite of overwhelming evidence that it's not the case.

This bias can also extend to how we understand the behavior of others. Instead of looking for what's good, we notice things that don't meet our high standards. Or based on our initial impression, we reject someone without giving them a fair chance.

Changing a negative view

Many years ago, I worked with a manager who was difficult to like. This woman would appear tender and kind-hearted, but then she would create rules that made my work life miserable. When she smiled during a conversation, I always worried she had a hidden agenda.

On the days when it was hardest to work with her, I allowed my negative feelings to come out. I expressed disagreement with her judgments and I complained about how her policies were affecting the staff.

But one day, I decided to turn my negative appraisal into compassion. I noticed that many of her actions came because she was trying to please her own boss. I began to see her loneliness and her great desire to be liked. I realized that my saying negative things about her to other staff members had further complicated my ability to work with her.

When I began to show compassion to this manager, our work relationship took a positive turn. I started asking more about her life and I volunteered to help more with projects. I also realized she was trying to accomplish organizational goals, not make me unhappy. In this case, showing compassion required grace and forgiveness, but it changed that relationship and improved my attitude toward my work.

Compassionate acts such as giving someone a compliment or assisting with a task can help you overcome your negative bias toward that person. This also helps you approach others with a sense of grace and forgiveness.

With difficult people, you might speak a few words of appreciation or ask how they are doing. In many cases, you may not hear positive feedback or even a "thank you." But your goal is to express compassion, regardless of the response you receive.

Andrew Dreitcer with the Center for Engaged Compassion believes that working with a difficult person demands more of our empathy. He recommends asking ourselves these questions:

- What could this person be fearing?
- What does this person long for?
- What emotional wounds might this person be living with?
- What cry of suffering can you imagine this person is making?
- What does this person need most?

If your negative viewpoints get in the way of showing compassion, you might need to re-train your thinking.

Here are three simple steps to help you do this:

Step 1. Demonstrate compassion for yourself.

Start by considering what you need the most right now. Perhaps you yearn for a few calm moments, a space that is safe and relaxing, or someone to be kind to you. Think about how you could meet some of these needs. Then do a few things that demonstrate compassion toward your own self.

Step 2. Think about someone in your life who is easy to care about.

This might be a person or even a pet. Do a small act of kindness that demonstrates the kind of compassion you want yourself.

3. Now extend your actions to someone who is harder for you to care about.

Choose a small act of compassion that feels safe and requires only a little courage. Perhaps leave an extra tip for your server at a restaurant. Or offer someone a ride to the doctor's office or physical therapy.

By doing a few small acts of compassion, you'll be able to move past your negative view of the world. And in the process, you'll probably find you become much happier and content with your life.

CHAPTER 8

Self-Compassion

YOU COULD ALWAYS COUNT on Carol. She was routinely there with comfort and caring whenever there was a need. In our church family, she was the first one to show up with flowers or baked goods when someone had surgery or an illness. It seemed that everyone loved her, and many people spoke of how kind and helpful Carol had been to them.

Yet when I got to know her, Carol told me about her constant struggles with anxiety and low-grade depression. She always wanted to be accepted and approved by others, and she worried about what people thought about her.

She told me she felt like an impostor in relationships because she believed if others could see her flaws, they wouldn't like her. When she excelled at a task, she would quickly point out the one small detail she didn't get right. She was wonderful at displaying compassion for others, but she couldn't do the same for herself.

Lack of self-compassion

You may believe harsh self-criticism will help you become a better person, but instead, it promotes negative emotions that drag you down. It also prevents you from achieving the kind of self-improvement you want so much.

In the book *The Kindness Cure*, Tara Cousineau says that self-criticism does not promote positive change; it only keeps us stuck.

When Jesus was asked about the most important principle of life, he responded, "Love your neighbor as yourself." We think this tells us to love our neighbors, so we try to do that. But unfortunately, we often don't get past the first half of that sentence. Jesus makes the point that you must love *both* your neighbor and yourself. And if you don't cultivate self-compassion, you will struggle more with loving your neighbor.

We tend to ignore the part about loving yourself because we equate it with traits we dislike. We worry that we'll be selfish, self-centered or unkind. But self-compassion doesn't involve any of these negative traits. Instead, it requires treating yourself with kindness, caring, understanding and patience.

When I reflect on my life decisions, both good and bad, I remind myself that I always did the best I could at that time. In hindsight, I might have chosen a different path or made wiser choices. But at the moment of a decision, I didn't have the same knowledge, skills or insight that I do now. So berating myself about a "bad" decision doesn't serve any purpose.

What did I learn?

Rather than treat ourselves harshly about life choices, we need to view ourselves as learners. Ask yourself, "What did I learn from this situation?" or "What would I do differently now that I am wiser?"

These learning moments will have a more positive impact on our lives than berating ourselves for decisions made when we had insufficient understanding or experience. They also help us allow for imperfections and acknowledge that we don't know everything.

Self-compassion enables us to calm our inner critic and live life with greater courage. Instead of self-criticism, you can

CHAPTER 8: SELF-COMPASSION

create a different story by reminding yourself, "Some things happened that I hadn't counted on. I will do better next time." Or you can say, "Now I know more about what I'm capable of as well as what I need to work on."

Sociologist Brené Brown encourages people to view themselves with kindness. She says, "We are often our own worst critics. We talk to ourselves in ways that we would never speak to someone else. With self-compassion, we can learn to understand and calm our inner critic, which is key to living a brave life."

In her book *The Gifts of Imperfection*, Brown says, "When we're kind to ourselves, we create a reservoir of compassion that we can extend to others."

Focusing on grace, rather than judgment

When I was a teenager, an older pastor at our church asked me to help him with Sunday communion. I was hesitant and told him, "I don't know if I should because I haven't done it before. What if I get it wrong?"

He encouraged me to give it a try. Then he explained that I would walk along the altar, break off pieces of bread from a loaf and hand them out to the people who were communing. He would follow behind me giving out the individual cups of wine.

After several passes down the row, I noticed I was leaving a trail of breadcrumbs, much like Hansel and Gretel. At the end of one row, I quietly said to the pastor, "Look at the mess I'm making. What will people say?"

He whispered, "They'll just say you're crummy." That was exactly what I needed to hear. I laughed and never worried about it again. I loved how that pastor focused on grace, not criticism or judgment.

We might easily show grace to others but find it hard to show it to ourselves. Grace allows for flaws, giving us a chance to get it right the next time. It gives us room to sometimes say and do things imperfectly. Grace helps us know we don't have to be perfect to be okay. It also builds stronger self-compassion that improves our ability to care about others.

Forgive past failures

All of us have had times when we "failed" at something. Maybe it was a school exam or a job interview. If you've ever been fired from a job, you might have concluded that it was your fault because of your work failures.

There can be times when negligence or a poor work style contributed to losing your job. But if you dig deeper, you'll often find a manager or supervisor who had their own problems. Work or relationship "failures" usually involve more than just you. So let go of being hard on yourself and give yourself grace and forgiveness.

Self-compassion involves letting go of the past—a place you no longer live. It can mean giving up regrets for events you had no control over or relationships that didn't work out.

When you engage in compassionate understanding of your past, focusing on what went right rather than your failures, you discover how to let go of your mistakes and move on with your life.

When you can't let go

For many years, my wife ran a weight-loss clinic that focused on emotional and psychological issues. In many cases, people's struggles were connected to holding onto anger, bitterness or grief. Over time, these emotions make it hard to be caring and nurturing to ourselves. Until people are willing to let go of those feelings, they will struggle to find success in many areas of their lives.

Here is one of her client's stories:

Donna lived in a beautiful condo on the 20th floor of a high-rise building. One morning, her husband took the dog for a walk and never came back. After several hours, Donna called the police and over the next three days, officers searched for her husband but couldn't find any clues to where he might be. It seemed that Donna's husband had simply disappeared along with the dog that was her best friend.

But it got worse. A couple days later, Donna tried to withdraw money at an ATM machine but her debit card was declined. A bank officer informed her that both her checking and savings accounts were empty and tellers couldn't trace the withdrawals.

Within months, Donna was forced to declare bankruptcy and move to a new home. But six months after he disappeared, the husband was found in another town, living with a woman who had once been Donna's good friend.

For the next couple years, Donna was consumed by anger and bitterness. Her health began to suffer and she gained a lot of weight. Even though she was physically miserable, she couldn't bring herself to exercise or eat healthy foods.

When Donna came to my weight-loss clinic, I saw a formerly happy and successful woman who had been destroyed by her life events. As her tears fell, she told me, "I just can't get over what he did to me." But her anguish kept her from self-care and moving forward in her life.

At one of our meetings, I asked her, "How long do you want to hold on to your anger and bitterness about him? A month? A year? For the rest of your life?"

She answered, "I don't know how long but I'm not ready to let it go yet." When she left my office, I gave her an assignment. By our next visit, she was to give me an answer to that question.

At our meeting the following week, Donna told me she had thought about the question for days. Then she announced, "I don't want to hold on to those feelings any more at all. I am ready now, and I want to let it all go."

At that point, I gave her a piece of paper and asked her to write down the specific things she wanted to let go of. She wrote down, "My husband, my dog, my friend, and the pain this has caused for me."

When she finished writing, I asked her to crumple the piece of paper in her fist and squeeze it tightly. Then I said, "When you are ready to let go of everything on your list, open your hand and let the crumpled paper fall to the floor."

At that point, Donna froze. "I can't do it!" she said. "I thought I was ready, but I can't seem to open my hand."

I responded, "We will sit here together until you can let it go." So we sat, and we talked, and she cried, but her fist stayed closed. Twenty minutes went by and it was time for her to leave, but she still held the paper in her hand.

So I gently said, "It looks like you have a different answer to the question, and you want to hold onto your pain a bit longer." Suddenly she shouted, "No! I don't want to hold it any more!" At that point, she opened her hand and let the crumpled paper fall to the floor.

Then she stood up, hugged me, and said, "What a relief! Now I can start taking care of myself again."

Donna still had to do a lot of healing work, but she started back on her plan for healthy eating and exercise. When I saw her a year later, she had reached her goal weight and was walking three miles every day. She had also started volunteering at a center for abused women and loved being able to care about them.

Once Donna's self-compassion was restored, she was able to show compassion for others again, which led her to a happier, more contented life.

A positive outlook

Neuroscience shows that dwelling on something you did "wrong" keeps firing the neural pathways that support anxiety or feelings of hopelessness. In contrast, approaching life with a positive outlook supports the energizing pathways of your brain and promotes greater self-confidence.

Your mind will usually follow your body. If you stand tall, speak calmly and walk with energy in your step, you are more likely to feel mentally strong and positive. Research tells us that positive thinkers tend to have a greater sense of self-worth and more ability to adapt to life's challenges.

For many years, one of my greatest support people was a white-haired saint named Elisa. She was one of my church members who remained kind and encouraging during one of the most challenging times in my career.

Elisa never showed judgment or criticized people around her. Instead, she invited us to family dinners and provided a safe and inviting place for visits and holiday gatherings. She also had an amazing ability to stay positive no matter what was going on.

When I sat down to talk about my problems, she'd say, "It will all be okay. You'll manage it or you'll find a better way to do things." Over and over, she would tell me, "It will all work out. Just hang in there and everything will be fine." Her confidence was contagious and I would walk away saying to myself, "Of course I can do this."

Elisa's positive outlook on life remained strong until her death at age 98. I feel so blessed to have known Elisa and I cherish her many lessons and the way her self-compassion helped so many people.

Self-compassion and life satisfaction

If you struggle with feeling unhappy or dissatisfied in life, you might consider changing some of your old messages and self-beliefs. Self-compassion acknowledges our shortcomings but doesn't obsess over them or exaggerate them.

Roy Bennett, author of *The Light in the Heart*, says, "Accept yourself, love yourself, and keep moving forward. If you want to fly, you have to give up what weighs you down."

View life as an adaptive adventure where you learn from your struggles or failures. Perhaps you are taking on too much in your life. Or you believe a bad event or era in life has defined who you are.

During my teaching years, I developed a friendship with a guy named Ben. At first, I didn't know why he acted strange or didn't respond well to my questions. Then he told me that he suffered from epilepsy. There were days when I could tell he was slow of speech or awkward in mannerisms.

However, at the supermarket where he worked as a checkout clerk, Ben became known as the go-to person. He was kind and patient with all of his customers as well as the people he worked with. For most of his adult life, Ben was the captain and manager for a community softball team. He also cared for his aging parents and took them to medical appointments.

Ben seemed to always know when someone had a need, and through his kind and gentle spirit, he readily showed compassion. He worked at being a strong, healthy person, and he did not allow his physical condition to define his life.

Monitor self-talk

What you say to yourself can make or break nearly everything you do. Phrases such as "I can't do anything right" or "I'm such a failure" don't inspire you to change your patterns. In fact, these devaluing statements and half-truths usually push you further away from self-compassion

The opposite is also true. When you tell yourself "Come on, you are capable of doing anything!" you can almost guarantee you'll accomplish your goals.

Jack Canfield, co-author of the *Chicken Soup for the Soul* series, taught a unique way to change negative self-talk. In his workshops, he would encourage participants to counter negative messages by saying, "No matter what you say or do to me, I am still a worthwhile person!"

Then he would yell insults at the group, saying phrases such as, "You're fat" or "You're ugly" or "You never do anything right." Each time he said one of these lines, the participants had to respond by shouting back the "worthwhile person" sentence.

Self-compassion begins with mentally contradicting the negative messages you hear from others around you. So if your boss says you messed up on a report, you can listen and determine how you need to change it. At the same time, you can quietly remind yourself that you are always a worthwhile person.

Reframe the situation

When you reframe an event or a thought, you view it from a different perspective. The word "reframing" simply refers to changing the way you think or speak about something. For example, if it rained when you were planning a picnic, you could reframe your disappointment by saying, "This is great. Now I don't have to worry about bugs or getting dirt in my food." Or you could view the rain as a welcome excuse to curl up in your favorite chair with a good book.

If you struggle with self-compassion, reframing negative messages will help you see yourself differently. When you reframe a situation or an idea, you don't deny its existence; you simply take a fresh view toward it and invent a new message.

Whenever an old thought causes you to feel down about yourself, turn it into a positive statement by saying, "That's not true! Actually...," then fill in the sentence with a new ending.

For example, when you catch yourself thinking, "I can't do anything right," reframe it by saying, "That's not true! Actually I do lots of things extremely well." And when failure thoughts sneak in, reframe them by saying, "Actually, I'm not a failure. I am successful at many things." Then write a list of some of your successes such as raising your children, holding a job or baking a chocolate layer cake.

By reframing what you say to yourself, you develop an encouraging, positive voice instead of putting yourself down. Your self-compassion will grow stronger through reframing the negative situations in your life.

CHAPTER 9

Receiving Compassion

WE USUALLY THINK of compassion as a gift for someone else. We might show compassion to improve someone's life or to ease another's suffering. Other times, we use compassion as a simple way to care about people.

But how do you handle times when someone shows compassion for you and your needs? Do you find it hard to receive compliments or generosity? Ideally, you will respond to receiving compassion by showing appreciation and gratitude. But sometimes we struggle with doing this and we minimize compassionate acts.

For example, when someone says, "You did a good job on that project," you might feel embarrassed and say, "Oh, it was nothing." But in this case, you reject the affirmation. Or a friend gives you a compliment such as, "What a nice dress," and you respond negatively by saying, "This old thing? I don't like how it fits me." In these cases, people are being affirming and you are turning it down.

What about times when someone shovels the snow off your walk or fixes a squeaky door? Perhaps friends bring you flowers or a meal after you've had surgery. It's easy to depreciate these gifts by responding with comments such as, "Oh, you shouldn't have," or "You didn't need to do that."

Sometimes, we struggle with receiving compassion because we don't want to appear weak or needy. Maybe we feel embarrassed because it looks like we couldn't do something ourselves. We want to protect our self-image of being strong and capable. Perhaps you shift the compassion by pointing to others you believe are more deserving of help or praise.

Building the happy life you want requires countering old messages about not being good enough or not being worth someone's praise. You are not being selfish when you graciously accept compliments from others or respond with appreciation for someone's kindness.

Appreciating compassion

At the end of completing my Ph.D. program at the University of Denver, I faced the committee where I had to defend my research and writing. I had studied the field of communication for five years and invested many painful hours finishing my dissertation.

I had also been blessed to have six wonderful faculty members support and guide me in my work. Along the way, they had all given me many gifts of understanding and compassion.

At the completion of the "oral defense" of my work, the smiling committee members offered congratulations for a job well done. I knew that from this moment on, my life would be different.

But I realize now how much I failed at receiving their praise. I felt awkward and even embarrassed. I said things like, "There are several things I could have done better. I know I should have worked more on some sections of it." As these esteemed professors extolled the quality of my work, I didn't know how to graciously receive and appreciate their words.

I learned a lot from that experience and have tried to be more accepting when others show me attention or compassion. When I retired from my full-time faculty position at Regis

University, the dean of my department arranged for 30 of my colleagues to participate in my farewell party.

One by one, my friends and co-workers spoke about what they appreciated about my work at the university. Tears filled my eyes and my heart was full as I listened to their kind words and accolades. Unlike my experience at my dissertation defense, this time I found the words to warmly receive and appreciate their compassion for me.

Changing your view

You might be tempted to blame your lack of emotional response to compassion on your family upbringing. We know that childhood experiences influence the ways we express emotions. But they don't have to affect how we respond as adults. We all have the capacity to appreciate our past but also establish new directions for ourselves.

Rick Hansen, author of *Hardwiring Happiness*, describes how our brain circuitry tends to hold on to negative memories and forget the positive ones. To counter this negative bias, he suggests that we focus more on positive moments in life. Ultimately, this can help wire our brain for happiness.

In your life of giving and receiving compassion, remember to notice and appreciate kindness from others. You have to be willing to allow people to honor you, do nice things for you and care for you. When someone does an act of compassion for you, let that person know how much it means to you.

Savor the moments

In order to receive compassion from others, you might need to slow down and notice their efforts. Awaken your sense of wonder and let the "wow" moments linger in your experiences.

Consider how wonderful it is that someone values you enough to want to be a blessing in your life.

Fred Bryant, a social psychologist at Loyola University, describes appreciating compassionate acts as "savoring." Just as we savor the sunset, the giggling of a young child or the cuddling of a loved one, we can savor the moments when someone shows us compassion.

You can do this by talking about their actions and saving them in your memory bank. Go ahead and bask in the moment, marveling at the miracle of others who show such caring.

For me, this can be as simple as my wife bringing me a cup of coffee on a tired morning. That small step helps me adjust to the day. In this case, not much is said, but the appreciation is there. I make sure I respond with a smile and a simple, "Thank you."

Compassion when it's needed most

In 2010, my wife was diagnosed with breast cancer. She went through major surgery, but because her cancer was early stage, she didn't need to have chemotherapy or radiation. But for those of us who spend a lot of time showing compassion to others, it can be hard to let people show it to us. In looking back at that painful time of our lives, we both discovered the importance of receiving compassion.

Here is Linda's story:

Learning I had breast cancer was awful. But what happened next amazed me and helped me get through my treatment and recovery.

On the day after I received the diagnosis, I called my sister as well as two of my best friends. They responded perfectly. They were horrified. Shocked. Sad for me. But their words were only part of my comfort. It was their actions that spoke the most.

Within a few hours of my telephone call, one friend brought over a small square white box. Inside was a beautiful print scarf, the huge kind that you can wrap around in a knot and wear with a sweater. It was my favorite colors, with lots of purple and teal. From the minute I looked at it, I felt stronger and more confident I could face what was ahead. If nothing else, I knew I could stay colorful!

Later that day, another friend came to my door with a loaf of freshly baked cinnamon bread, still warm from her oven. We immediately sat down and ate a few slices, giving us a sense of connection as well as great comfort.

My sister was on a plane within days and stayed with me for a week. She sat with my husband during my surgery, then helped take care of me as I recovered. She went with me to the stores that carried special mastectomy bras and stood with me while I learned about wigs and scarves to wear during chemo. Her presence helped me feel less alone as I dealt with the fears and the treatment steps.

After my double mastectomy surgery, the initial pathology report came back showing the tumor was localized and had not spread. That meant I wouldn't need chemotherapy. But two days later, a revised report showed one lymph node had been positive, and my surgeon said that almost guaranteed I'd need both chemo and radiation.

I emailed my list of friends, and let them know it looked like I'd be having chemo after all. A few minutes after I sent the email, my doorbell rang. It was my friend holding another loaf of cinnamon bread. "I just read your email," she said, "and I am SO sorry!"

We hugged and we both cried. I was totally moved by her sensitive caring gesture. Someone knew I was in pain, and that was all that mattered. I loved how she responded so quickly to let me know that she cared.

About six weeks after my surgery, my oncologist informed me I wouldn't be needing chemo after all. Instead, I ended up taking one of the long-term drugs used to prevent cancer reoccurrence. I am blessed to be a "survivor" now for many years.

I learned a lot from having breast cancer. I learned that I could survive a very difficult time and that eventually, I would heal and recover. I also learned some amazing lessons on how to help a friend or family member diagnosed with cancer or a major illness. Of course, everyone responds differently, but based on my own experiences, here are some things I suggest:

- Respond quickly.
- Be shocked. Be sad. Be hopeful. Be all of them.
- Send an email or a card, or both.
- Call and ask when it's a good time to stop over.
- Or email, and ask when it's a good time to call.
- Ask which day you could deliver a meal. Use disposable pans.
- Send a gift card to a nearby restaurant. Offer to pick up a take-out order.
- Be a presence. Be willing to sit with and even cry with them. Be silent at times.

Show up with a token of some kind. I told you about the scarf and the bread. A different friend brought a gift bag that contained homemade scones, flavored teas and a special card. Another left off a stack of books, saying, "Don't worry about when you return these."

Before we learned I wouldn't need to have chemotherapy, one amazing friend offered to drive me to appointments and sit and read during my treatment. Others brought meals or offered to pick up food orders for us. I appreciated every one of these simple gifts. And receiving compassion from others gave me a deeper understanding of what it feels like to allow people to care.

Showing gratitude

When someone shows compassion or does something special for you, try to give back in some way. It may be as simple as a thank-you card, an appreciative email, or doing another act of kindness.

When our dog Peppy died, we received a lot of "loss of dog" sympathy cards. Most of them included handwritten notes expressing how hard it is to lose a deeply loved pet. People really seemed to understand our sadness, and they expressed how much they cared about us and our loss.

After taking all the cards down from our fireplace mantle, my wife sent a short email to each of the senders. With a subject of "Thank you for being our friend," she wrote, "I was going through the wonderful notes we received after Peppy died, and I wanted you to know how much we loved your card and kind words. We appreciated you caring about us and being a friend when we really needed it."

Acknowledging the cards and messages gave us a chance to show we appreciated receiving compassion. Of course, losing a dog is nothing compared to the death of a loved one or family member. But if you go through any kind of loss, open your heart to receiving caring and kindness. And if possible, respond by letting those who showed compassion know how much you appreciated their words and actions.

Appreciate caring people

After a hurricane a couple years ago, a church disaster team spent a week clearing debris from the yards of many homeowners. At the end of their stay, the exhausted workers went out to dinner together. When the team leader went to pay for their meals, the cashier said, "Your bill has been paid by someone who appreciates your gift of service."

What a beautiful way to give back to those who have showed compassion. Watch for times when you can respond to an act of kindness, even ones as small as someone holding a door or picking up the note you dropped. A simple "thank you" shows gratitude to the person who helped you.

In his research with more than a thousand people, University of California professor Robert Emmons found that those who live with a life orientation of gratitude tend to possess higher levels of positive emotions. They have more joy in their lives, more optimism and greater connection to other people.

Gratitude notices the "wow moments" of compassion and uses them to celebrate what is good in life. It also validates the people who show you caring and kindness. When my wife shops for groceries, she usually asks the name of the clerk who does the check-out. When she leaves, she calls that person by name and thanks them for their work. This seems like such a simple response, but the clerks always smile and appreciate her comments.

Whenever you are on the receiving end of an act of compassion, make an effort to show your gratitude. It will help you feel more positive and joyful in your day.

CHAPTER 10

Compassion in Communities

DURING MY SEMINARY YEARS in St. Paul, Minnesota, I worked part-time at a nursing home. In addition to doing physical care, I spent time talking to the residents and tried to show kindness whenever I could.

In a room at the end of a long hallway lived a delightful 85-year-old woman named Sophie. During one of my stops to see her, I noticed several books on her bedside stand, so I asked her about them.

She explained that she had been a schoolteacher most of her life, and the books reminded her of how much she enjoyed reading with her students. Then I asked, "Would you like me to read to you?" With a big smile, she said, "I would love that!"

So during my work days, I made sure to spend time with Sophie and read to her from her books. As she thanked me each time, she always looked so happy. She brought joy to my life as well because, you see, Sophie was blind.

In his book *Compassion*, theologian Henri Nouwen points out that compassion is a communal activity. It's an attitude and a way of life. It reveals itself in how we talk to each other and how we treat others. He reminds us that as compassionate people, we are not neutral about the suffering of others. Instead, he encourages us to be passionate as we watch for opportunities to care about people.

Think about all the places where you are part of a group or community. You probably go to work, take kids to school or attend church. You might spend time with family members and friends and perhaps participate in neighborhood events.

In all of these communities, people long to be valued and cared about, and acts of compassion provide a wonderful way to demonstrate this. Sometimes, we need to slow down and take time to listen or do things for others. Even the busiest setting can still be a place to show compassion.

Compassion in schools

Regardless of your age, being in school can feel scary and even unsafe. We live in an age when bullying happens a lot, and many kids struggle to get through the day without being harmed.

In Colorado, we lived close to a school that had classrooms for elementary students on the first floor and ones for junior high students on the second floor. For some years, the school challenged the older students to watch during recess for problems and protect the younger students from harm. Over time, students of all ages became friends, and bullying was almost nonexistent. This amazing school promoted a culture of kindness and caring among the students as well as the staff.

For parents, it can be difficult to get younger kids to talk about their school day. When you ask the typical question, "How was your day?" you'll probably hear, "Fine." But sometimes you want to know more, and it can be challenging to pull more answers from your child.

When our nieces and nephews were in school, we learned a new approach that worked every time. Since we didn't see them very often, we wanted to hear more details about their school days.

We would start by finding a convenient time, and then we would sit down and say, "Walk me through your day." Starting with how they got to school, we had them describe all of the parts of their school experience.

Usually we would prompt them by asking about the first class or period of the day. Then we would have them tell what they were studying, the name of the teacher, if they liked the class or the teacher and what they liked best about that topic. We learned amazing details that we wouldn't have heard if we had only asked, "How was your day?" We discovered how one sixth grade teacher made math a fun subject. Another teacher brought history alive by telling stories about the families of soldiers during famous wars.

We continued doing this when the kids were in college and found they still loved having us listen to stories about their classes and relationships. These talks built long-lasting connections that we still enjoy today.

With younger kids, you won't want to push for this much detail every day. But walking through your child's day once a week or even once a month might give you fresh insights about how school is going. You might also begin to notice learning or social struggles that need some attention.

The need for a compassionate school community stays with us throughout life. One of my favorite professors in graduate school had a messy office. He had books stacked all around, and his desk was usually covered with papers to read and lists of phone messages. But somehow, he always made time for me.

When I came in and started complaining about school, he would always pull out a chair and tell me to sit down. Then he would look me in the eye and say, "Tell me what's going on."

I loved how he valued me and treated me as the most important person in his day. His compassion helped me through many tough times while I completed my studies. I felt so proud to see him on the platform when I received my doctorate degree.

Compassion where you don't expect it

A few months ago, I was extra tired, so I went to Perkins, one of my favorite restaurants, for breakfast. My server treated me well, brought my food quickly and even asked about how I was doing that morning. As she turned and started walking away, I saw the back of her shirt which read, "Kindness served here."

The timing couldn't have been better. The server's kindness and attention perked me up and helped me feel positive about life again. Before I left, I told her how much her compassion had meant to me. And I loved this example of a corporation striving to create a caring atmosphere for both guests and employees.

You may not have any power over the culture at your workplace. But you can certainly become a culture-of-one who strives to make a difference in people's lives. In fact, one person's compassion for forgotten people can be enough to ignite a flame of caring in an entire community.

Kaylee Ciavarelli's grandmother had dementia and lived in a nursing home in Iowa. Whenever she visited her grandmother, Kaylee felt a lot of empathy for the her as well as the other patients who had Alzheimer's and dementia.

She turned that empathy into compassion with a doll project. Through a fundraising effort, Kaylee purchased realistic looking dolls that could be held and cuddled by nursing home residents. She called them Dola Dolls, named after her grandmother Dola.

She was amazed at how the dolls helped uplift people's spirits. She said, "Residents who weren't talking before are now smiling at their babies and singing Happy Birthday along with the group."

Kaylee added, "Most women don't forget how to be nurturers. When they have that baby in their arms, you really see their nurturing side come out. It has decreased a lot of the tension in these patients and made them happier."

She continued, "They view them as real. My grandma would lay her baby down and put pillows around it so it wouldn't roll off the bed while she had lunch."

Kaylee's compassion for these patients has spread to other states and nursing home locations, and her dolls are being used in many other places. The residents have usually been delighted to give the dolls a home and serve as their caregivers.

Unknown problems

A couple years ago, I was asked to consult at a health center that did medical testing, education and treatment for diabetic patients. The work schedules began early most mornings and often ran into evening hours. But fatigue, high levels of stress and relationship issues were taking a toll on the staff members.

When I met with the group, I began with reviewing the mission and values of the center and then did a few team-building exercises. Everyone seemed pleasant enough, but when we began talking about job responsibilities, the tension increased. The nurses were upset about the long hours and the difficulty of getting all of the required tasks done each day.

But they also talked about their frustration with staff members who weren't doing their share of the work. When I asked for specifics, the discussion centered on one nurse who apparently avoided early morning or evening appointments and some days relied on others to finish the day's work.

When I asked this staff member what was going on, she began to cry. Then she quietly shared that she had never told the staff, but she was attending Alcoholics Anonymous meetings in the early mornings and some evenings. She said, "I've been sober now for two years, but it's still so hard. Most days, I'm just trying to keep my life together."

The other nurses immediately responded with an outpouring of empathy and a willingness to support her in this personal battle. They worked out a different schedule and reassigned some of the daily tasks to other staff members.

Over time, the nurse's performance improved, and she told the staff members how grateful she was for their support. This team created a compassionate community that made a difference in one nurse's life.

Compassion in neighborhoods

The neighborhoods where we live all have their own distinctive cultures. My wife grew up on a farm in the Midwest where neighbors knew each other well and were quick to show compassion. When a farmer became ill or was injured, others jumped in to care for livestock or harvest crops.

These days, many people live in crowded apartment buildings or communities where neighbors don't even know each other's names. But when disaster strikes, you'll often see an amazing neighborhood response as people try to help those around them.

In the past few years, we have seen forest fires burn millions of acres of trees along with thousands of homes and businesses. Hurricanes have damaged homes, caused major flooding and disrupted home life.

But in the midst of those disasters, we've read moving stories about people who quickly showed up with chain saws to cut away fallen trees blocking streets and roads. Other times, we've learned about food and clothing drives for people who lost everything in a fire.

When we had a big snowstorm last year, I was dreading going out into the cold and clearing the snow drifts from my driveway and sidewalk. But when I looked out the window, I saw that my neighbor had already shoveled the snow from both her own driveway and mine. That act of compassion meant so much to me and reminded me to watch for opportunities to do similar things for others.

Compassion grows

You might think your acts of compassion are too small to matter or make a difference. But often your caring spirit will inspire others to show compassion as well. And sometimes that can build until it affects thousands.

In 2017, the University of Iowa opened a new Children's Hospital that overlooks the university's football field, Kinnick Stadium. A football fan named Krista Young was inspired by photos of the huge hospital and how it served so many sick children and their families.

She realized that from an area on the 12th floor of the hospital, some of the patients could see everyone in the football stands and wave to them. On a whim, she thought it would be great if the fans waved back. She shared her idea with Levi Thompson who managed a Facebook page for Iowa Hawkeye football fans.

Levi loved her idea and throughout the summer, he added lots of photos of the hospital and the view from the top. Then he posted a request for fans to turn and wave between the first and second quarters of the next game. By the day of the home opener, his posts had earned more than two million views, so he had a good feeling about this fun way to encourage the hospital patients.

Krista wasn't sure it would work, especially since the university had not promoted the wave or made any announcements about it at the end of the first quarter. She said, "I assumed groups here and there might do it." But she watched in total amazement when all 70,000 fans turned toward the hospital, raised their arms and waved to the children.

Since that first time, the University of Iowa wave continues to happen at the end of the first quarter at every home game. At night games, the wave is done with flashlights on cell phones. All of the players and fans pause for a minute to honor the patients at the hospital, many of whom are extremely ill.

The patients and families call this "a wave of hope" and "life-changing." While social media helped make this campaign a success, it also shows the power of responding to that quiet inner voice that urges us toward a small act of compassion.

CHAPTER 11

Compassion in Organizations

NINE PEOPLE STOOD in a circle in the front yard of an elderly man whose home had been damaged by a severe wind storm. For the past four days, these volunteers had cut down huge trees and moved the limbs to the curb. They'd covered holes in the roof with plastic tarps, cleaned up huge piles of debris and provided disposable coolers for storing perishable foods until the electricity came back on.

As part of a recovery team with Missouri Baptist Disaster Relief, these individuals were ready to move to the next home assigned by their leader. But before they left, they stood quietly and prayed for healing and protection for George, the homeowner. Then the leader stepped forward and gave George a new Bible. On the blank pages inside the back cover, the team members had each written personal notes and signed their names.

With tears running down his face, George accepted their gift and in a broken voice thanked them for what they had done. He told them, "I was so devastated by this storm and I had no idea what I was going to do. I am a widower and don't have any family close by. Your kindness helped me find back my spirit and my reason to live. I will treasure this Bible and read it every day."

My brother-in-law, Dave, was one of the members of this group. Since he retired a few years ago, he has gone on dozens of trips with this organization and has helped clean up after floods, hurricanes and tornadoes. The team members usually sleep on church floors and use the bathrooms and showers in the specially equipped semi-trucks brought to the disaster area.

He told me, "Our motto is Help, Hope and Healing. So beside the physical labor, we talk to the homeowners, listen a lot and share the gospel. When we do our prayer circle and give the homeowners a Bible at the end of a job, we all get pretty emotional."

Dave said many of the homeowners will ask how they can pay us back for our work. He said, "Our response is always the same. We tell them that it's already paid because Jesus has paid the debt for them."

During a typical year, this group does disaster trips many times. Dave says, "Helping others through difficult times becomes a blessing to us as well as those who we serve."

When disasters happen

Many churches and local organizations are known for being on the front lines after natural disasters. Their volunteers work tirelessly to help with recovery from the hardest losses anyone could imagine. From these acts of service and compassion, they hear amazing stories of gratitude and changed lives.

In August of 2020, a major storm called a derecho tore through central Iowa. In just over 45 minutes, high winds and torrential rain destroyed buildings, tore holes in roofs and toppled 200-year-old trees. In Cedar Rapids, thousands of people lost electricity, some for more than ten days.

Within hours of the storm, churches, Army Reserve units, and groups such as the Salvation Army mobilized to help people who were injured or trapped in their damaged homes.

Hugh semi-trucks rolled into town bringing portable kitchens, bathrooms and showers.

Over the next few weeks, volunteers cleared trees from blocked streets, delivered coolers filled with food to stranded residents and transported hundreds of people to safer locations. Day after day, our TV and online news gave updates on the progress in the recovery from the derecho. But in addition to showing piles of debris and ruined homes and cars, they interviewed people who expressed tremendous gratitude for the help they had received.

In one condominium development, homeowners who had a working gas stove gave out gallons of hot water for coffee every morning. During the ten days without electricity, their neighbors said that having cups of hot coffee became one of the best gifts shared during the recovery.

In another neighborhood, a resident who owned a generator ran long extension cords to several homes. Then neighbors took turns using the generator to run freezers and refrigerators to protect food and medications. During their turns with having electricity, some people cooked extra food and shared it with neighbors around them.

After a disaster, these acts of compassion make a huge difference in helping people cope during recovery. They also connect strangers and bring healing and support when it's needed most.

Organizations that demonstrate compassion

I have been fortunate to never go hungry. I will admit that, as a child, I sometimes got tired of eating hot dogs or canned soup. But even though I complained about my food, I never went to school on an empty stomach.

In our current world, troubled home situations and lack of money have increased food insecurity for thousands of children as well as adults. The term "food insecurity" is defined as the lack of regular access to safe and nutritious food. This causes many children to go to school hungry, which harms their focus and makes learning difficult.

Fortunately, there are many compassionate organizations that are helping with these challenges as well as many other needs. When you research these groups, you'll find ongoing requests for donations, volunteers and financial support.

In your own steps toward doing more compassionate acts, I urge you to consider offering help where you can. You can find hundreds of organizations who would gladly accept your kindness and financial help.

Here are several organizations that provide wonderful help and support to those in need:

Food banks and food pantries

These nonprofit organizations provide low-cost food options for those who need it most. Food banks tend to be larger places that collect and distribute food to hunger-related organizations such as local food pantries.

For most kids, school lunches provide food during the week. But on weekends and holidays, many homes have little food available. To help remedy this, many churches and other organizations offer backpack food programs. Volunteers fill small backpacks with nutritious, nonperishable, easy-to-prepare meals and snacks to help children deal with not having enough food at home.

These groups are always seeking volunteers to work in their centers. They also accept donations of many types of food and supplies.

Disaster relief organizations

Most of you are familiar with the bell ringers and red kettles you see around the holidays each year. But you probably have no idea where all the money collected goes. With the red kettle donations as well as major fundraising events throughout the year, the Salvation Army provides help for dozens of major areas.

The Salvation Army's website proclaims, "We fight nature's fury with human kindness." And it demonstrates this through not only major disaster relief, but also dozens of other programs, including homeless shelters, programs for veterans, rehabilitation, and help for domestic abuse.

The American Red Cross also jumps in when there's a natural disaster. Volunteers from this organization are usually first on the scene after a house fire, providing emergency shelter, food, clothing and financial assistance. But they also respond quickly to help people after major disasters such as hurricanes, flooding, tornadoes and earthquakes. All of the disaster assistance is free, which is made possible by voluntary donations of time and money.

Many other organizations such as Samaritan's Purse, as well as teams from churches and schools, offer immediate help to people affected by a natural disaster. Nearly all of these services are provided by volunteers.

Habitat for Humanity

This global housing organization has helped millions of struggling people be able to live in a real home. Habitat's vision is for a world where everyone has a decent place to live. Using volunteers as well as the future Habitat homeowners, this organization builds affordable, decent homes for people who need them the most.

Habitat for Humanity is not a giveaway program. In addition to making mortgage payments, homeowners invest 500 volunteer hours into the building of their homes and the homes of others. By partnering with the potential homeowners, Habitat helps build strength, stability and self-reliance that go beyond owning a home.

Two of the most dedicated workers with Habitat are former President Jimmy Carter and former first lady Rosalynn Carter. Throughout their involvement with Habitat, they have become tireless advocates, active fundraisers, and some of the organization's best hands-on construction volunteers.

Jonathan Reckford, the CEO of Habitat for Humanity since 2005, has seen the powerful benefits of people from all walks of life working together to help one another. In his phenomenal book, *Our Better Angels*, he shares true stories of people involved with Habitat as volunteers and future homeowners.

Mr. Reckford believes that Habitat makes a powerful case for showing compassion. He says, "When we approach the world with an outward sense of giving rather than an inward sense of keeping our gifts to ourselves, we can face the toughest challenges from a place of peace."

The people you can't see

In all types of organizations, you can find opportunities to show compassion, even to people who are "invisible" workers. You probably never see the staff member who empties the trash or cleans the bathrooms at your office.

Night-shift workers in manufacturing companies, hospitals and emergency response phone banks provide critical services. But sometimes, instead of being appreciated, these workers are criticized for not doing things "right."

Think about the people you rarely see who take care of your needs in life. That might include someone who opens another checkout line at the supermarket so you can get home sooner. At a restaurant, the kitchen crew members cook your meal, but you see only the worker who sets your food in front of you.

Sometimes, it's a challenge to show compassion to people you can't see. But I've been surprised at the stories I've heard about people who do that.

Many years ago, I was sent to the Naval Air Station in Japan on a short-term assignment as a chaplain. While I was on duty, we learned the Chief of Chaplains, a high-ranking admiral, was coming to the base for a visit. In the Navy, this was a big deal, so we quickly prepared for a formal visit and planned for him to meet with everyone who was important.

At the appointed time, with huge flags waving from each of the front fenders, the Chief's car approached the base. Everyone along the roadway saluted the car, and it was an impressive entry.

Since it was almost lunchtime when the Chief arrived, the senior staff invited him to accompany all of us to the Officers Club. He said, "No, we aren't going there. Instead, we will all go to the dining hall where the enlisted members have lunch."

We shuddered at the thought of an admiral walking through a dining hall where lower ranked sailors were eating. But based on his instructions, we took him to that area of the base.

As we picked up our trays and moved through the food line, the Chief disappeared. A few minutes later, we saw him wandering through the cooking area where he was shaking hands and telling people how much he valued their work. In his act of kindness, he honored the workers who are usually invisible, especially to high-ranking officers.

Compassion through listening

In many organizations, the governing board and influential staff members have the greatest say in day-to-day operations. However, inclusive groups find ways to give voice to those who otherwise may not be heard.

One company accomplished this by creating a "listening committee." This group's primary function is to hear complaints, innovative ideas, or feedback about how things were going.

A listening committee seeks feedback from all areas of the organization that might otherwise go unheard. It also gives team members a way to voice their preferences and concerns in a safe way.

At one university where I taught communication classes, some students complained about not having anyone to talk to when they were troubled. So the school set up a couple of areas on the campus to invite people to talk. They installed pairs of facing benches and put up signs that said, "Listening post. Talk here."

If students or staff members wanted to talk to someone, they would sit down on one of the benches. Usually within minutes, another person would join them and the visit would begin. Amazingly, these benches seemed to always have a couple people sitting on them and talking.

The visits might have lasted for only five minutes, but the one who needed to talk felt cared about because someone listened. The students loved it because it gave them a chance to connect with another person in a safe, nonthreatening way.

Don't be so stubborn

The International Charter for Compassion promotes repairing relationships everywhere, including those between feuding groups. Their charter proclaims:

We urgently need to make compassion a clear,
luminous and dynamic force in our polarized world.
Rooted in a principled determination to transcend
selfishness, compassion can break down political,
dogmatic, ideological and religious boundaries.

In my mediation work involving churches, I frequently encountered a well-meaning stubbornness that got in the way of relationships. Usually the stubborn people began to soften once they felt heard in respectful conversations.

Some years ago, I was asked to help mediate a dispute between a rabbi who was head of a Jewish community and the imam who served a large Muslim group. These two leaders had been arguing for some time over their differing views about serving their people.

Recently, they had started fighting in public through newspaper articles and radio shows. The men had each told their congregants to have nothing to do with people from the other religion, even if they were neighbors or friends. It became obvious that many people were getting hurt by this feud.

Because a national convention was scheduled to begin in a few months, the city planners worried about bad press. Based on their request, my colleague and I agreed to meet with the two men and see if we could help them get past their problems. Since neither of the men would go near the other's church, we had to find a neutral site for our meeting. We settled on a city library that was not used by either of their groups.

When we arrived at the meeting room, the two men sat at opposite ends of a 10-foot-long table. They were barely speaking to each other but answered our questions and talked about their anger toward each other.

This unique mediation lasted six weeks. At each meeting, we would listen to them describe their complaints and allow them to rant about their issues.

Eventually, the two agreed to do small acts of kindness such as returning each other's phone calls, coming to our meetings on time and showing respect in how they spoke to each other. The also decided they would each write one paragraph that said something good about the other and publish these in their organization's newsletter.

Finally, they made an agreement to discuss their differences of opinions in person before going to the press or radio station. Little by little, they began to resolve their conflicts.

When we finally reached a point where they were getting along, I asked them to stand up from the table, walk toward each other and shake hands. They cautiously approached each other, then reached out and shook hands. I saw tears in their eyes as they thanked us for helping them move past their anger and bitterness and rebuild this important relationship.

As we completed our meeting, I thanked them for working so hard on these challenging issues. Then I asked the men a final question, "Will you need any more help from us?" The rabbi said, "We're grown men. We can talk through issues on our own as they come up." The imam agreed.

When I spoke with the rabbi a few months later, he said they were doing great and were cooperating well with each other's groups. In this situation, a few small compassionate acts built a relationship that could not be envisioned at the beginning of our discussions.

CHAPTER 12

Compassion at Work

IN 2007, PETER MBONABUCHA fled his home in Burundi, Africa, and came to the United States where he became a citizen. In his efforts to build a new life, he studied English and took college classes in the field of medical education.

Peter also worked as a part-time cashier at a chain grocery store in my hometown in Iowa. Around 2:30 one afternoon, a customer who seemed rushed came through his line. When Peter told him the total for his groceries was $112, the customer became rather flustered and said he had only $100.

The man explained that because he was late for work, he had left home in a hurry that morning and forgotten his wallet. A work friend had loaned him $100 in cash so he could purchase food and supplies for a gathering of friends that evening. As he looked at his cart and tried to figure out which items to remove, Peter stepped from behind the counter and used his own debit card to pay the difference.

The customer thanked him and went on his way. But he wanted to do something more to show his appreciation, so he set up an online fundraiser titled "The $12 Impact," hoping to raise $1000. He also shared the story on Facebook, and by the end of one week, the fund had grown to more than $5000. He set up a plan with the grocery store manager to present an oversized mock-up check to Peter and he invited a TV news crew to film the story.

Peter was surprised by the event and said he didn't even remember helping that customer. He also shared that during his early years in the United States, he struggled with finances. He said, "One time when I ran out of money and couldn't pay for my groceries, somebody paid the rest of my bill. From that day on, I have tried to pay it forward and do good things for others who need help."

One person's compassion can make a significant difference in another person's life. It can also spark the light of compassion in others who see what we've done. Over the past several years, the "pay it forward" concept has caught on, and I've learned of many situations where someone took care of the next person in line at the coffee shop or even the gas station.

Please notice me

Because most of us spend a great deal of time at work, we long for a place where we feel noticed and cared about. We want to feel appreciated by our co-workers and valued by the leadership.

When people are interviewed about what they like about their work setting, the responses are frequently the same. People say, "My co-workers are kind and generous," or "This organization cares about the people who work here."

Of course, in many work settings, that isn't the typical style. But whether you are an employee, a leader or the owner of a company, you can contribute to a compassionate work culture.

Each time you show concern for a co-worker, you set up the potential for reciprocal actions. We know that when someone is helpful or shows us kindness, we tend to return the favor. Even small acts of compassion promote greater cooperation in our work relationships.

Kindness and thoughtfulness also encourage people to have greater flexibility and be more supportive in their work. In times of high stress, compassionate work relationships are the ones that most often come to our aid. We look out for our friends and whenever possible, help them get past challenges.

Sometimes kindness shows up when we least expect it. John Chambers was the CEO of the highly successful company Cisco Systems for nearly 20 years. During his time with the company, it grew from annual revenues of $70 million to more than $47 billion.

Chambers was known for his strong leadership style and successful sales approach. But very few people knew that from early childhood, he had struggled with dyslexia. Fortunately, he had worked with tutors who helped him learn how to work around this and manage it. He rarely talked about his reading challenges, but one year at a "take your child to work day," he got caught off guard.

In an interview with *Forbes*, he described what happened:

"I witnessed a young girl break down in tears after having trouble asking me questions. This girl said that she was dyslexic, and forgetting that my microphone was on, I said, 'I am too.'

"Then I told her, 'You have to picture what you want to do, take your time, memorize the concept rather than the question, and then just talk as if we are having a conversation.' From there, I suggested that she re-ask the question, and we went through it together.

"All of a sudden, the entire room was silent because, at the time, my dyslexia was a secret. I immediately worried that I had been too open because as a young and insecure CEO, I didn't want anyone to see my weaknesses. But since then, I've learned that many young CEOs have this same issue. I also believe the best leaders are candid about their strengths and weaknesses, and they are willing to speak openly about them."

Knowing that someone understands our situation becomes a small act of compassion. I'm sure the young girl never forgot that kind response from Mr. Chambers.

Please help me

Most of my co-workers knew that I am not friends with computers. I remember many days when my computer frustrated me to the point of anger. No matter what I tried, I couldn't get my computer to fix things or respond to my commands.

Fortunately, at my university job, I was in a compassionate work setting. Whenever I begged someone for help, I never heard, "I'm too busy." Even though it pulled people away from their own work, they came to my office and helped me figure things out. That kind of help always meant so much, and it enabled me to be successful at my job.

Some years ago, I was asked to help an international company deal with ongoing employee issues. Because the workers were dispersed at many sites around the world, coordinating their work was especially challenging. Their current project required operations managers to regularly call clients who worked in other countries.

Because of the time zone differences, Tim, who normally was a great employee, struggled to get his calls made. When his supervisor asked him why he was so far behind, Tim explained that his wife had just had a baby. She was physically exhausted and was struggling with the emotional challenges of being a new mother. Tim was working hard to help her, including spending many late nights up with the baby.

As we worked on ideas for helping the account managers, Tim's supervisor spoke up. He told Tim, "It's been many years ago for me now, but I've been there. Give me your list, and I'll make those late-night and early-morning calls. Right now, you need to take care of your wife."

Tim tearfully thanked his supervisor. Although Tim was a high performer at his job, his wife and newborn were also huge priorities for him. His supervisor's compassion helped him continue to do his job during this rough stretch of life.

Compassionate companies

We certainly understand the outcomes of showing compassion to individuals. But in work settings, compassion provides benefits for the entire company. Acts of kindness connect us to others in meaningful ways which then promote trust and cooperation. They also create resiliency by improving flexibility when employees deal with changing demands.

Whereas rigidity causes tension, flexibility builds strength. Compassion emphasizes a "we" attitude that supports teamwork and shared success. Because compassion addresses points of pain and responds to them, it builds a work setting that people want to belong to.

The well-known retailer Patagonia makes a large variety of athletic and outdoor clothing. But the company has also created an unconventional, one-of-a-kind culture. The employee handbook is titled, "Let My People Go Surfing," and supervisors readily allow workers to leave for a while when surf conditions are best.

Patagonia provides onsite childcare centers that include training in child development for new moms. It also offers a schedule option that gives workers a three-day weekend every other week. The goal of supporting employees at all levels has resulted in extremely high retention levels. People who work there want to stay!

Jane Dutton, a researcher at the University of Michigan, has studied an array of organizational settings including hospitals, universities and businesses. She found that when distressed employees received acts of compassion such as emotional support, time off from work, or even flowers, they showed more positive emotions such as joy and contentment. These employees also demonstrated greater commitment toward their work organizations.

But the research showed an interesting twist. These positive results existed whether employees received compassion directly or they merely witnessed it being shown to someone else.

Dutton encourages workers to pay attention to the psychological well-being of fellow employees and take action when needed. For example, if an employee experiences a loss such as a divorce or death in the family, she recommends that someone contact that employee within 24 to 48 hours and offer help.

Compassion is contagious

An issue of the journal *Emotion* describes an experiment in compassion at Coca Cola's headquarters in Madrid, Spain. For four weeks, University of California researchers looked at the impact of small acts of kindness on the business environment. These included sending thank-you notes, showing generosity, offering to help with demanding tasks, doing favors and expressing appreciation.

The researchers found that kind actions were contagious, and other workers began doing similar things. Soon the employees began to express greater satisfaction with work and a stronger feeling of camaraderie. In addition to being appreciated for their work, the employees loved being noticed and cared about.

I will never forget one of my own meaningful experiences with a company showing compassion. I was fairly new in my job at a university and was still learning about the work culture. When I arrived at my office one morning, I was surprised by the sight of hundreds of balloons festively placed in the halls and conference room. When one of the female employees arrived, she immediately received cheers from all of the gathered employees.

During the next few minutes, I learned that the festive event was not about promotions, achieving a department goal or a new hire. It was about the health of this worker and the team members were celebrating the ten-year anniversary of her being cancer-free. Tears ran down the worker's face as she saw the joy and love on the faces of this group of fellow employees.

Compassionate leadership

Scott Kriens is the chairman and former CEO of Juniper Networks, a highly successful technology company. During his years at the company, he saw it grow from a "handful of enthusiastic engineers" to a company of 7,500 people and $4 billion in sales worldwide. His key philosophy for success is that you have to start with the relationships among people.

He says, "The quality of the teams and their teammates is determined by the trust, the connection and the compassion they extend to each other." He believes we need to offer the benefit of the doubt during uncertainty, listen for understanding instead of disagreement, investigate assumptions and reflect on what is said by others. In essence, he says, "Be intentional about caring."

We often think of leaders as people who are assigned roles in a job or a company. However, leadership occurs in other ways that are just as important. Sharing your wisdom with a child is leadership. Calling your neighbor to tell him he left his garage door open is leadership.

For the past few years, I have worked as an election official for my local county government. When people show up to vote, this might appear to be an easy job. We verify people's identity, hand them a ballot and direct them to a voting booth.

But what voters can't see is the complex computer systems and the ever-changing election rules we have to follow. Often the workdays extend from 6 a.m. to 9 p.m. and during that time, we don't leave the building or our assigned location.

On election days, I have met a lot of compassionate leaders who made my work easier. Once when I was setting up a voting machine, I didn't understand some of the tasks and kept making mistakes. The group leader for the day patiently listened to me and then walked me through the steps again.

The computer programs we use for elections are frequently updated, and until I learned a new system, I would often make incorrect entries. Again, the leaders didn't make me feel incompetent. Instead, one of them would say, "Yes, that's hard to remember. Let's go over it again."

As I watched the skillful leaders on those workdays, I noticed they tended to be kind listeners, and they stayed affirming of our work in spite of things we got wrong. Even when faced with a line of impatient voters, the leaders always noticed my computer struggles and quickly helped me fix the problems. On those election days, I have been extra grateful for compassionate leadership.

Support staff as leaders

In work settings, leadership can be shown by a small act to help a colleague or a kind word to calm a co-worker's anxiety. Whatever the setting, compassionate leaders notice when someone is stressed or hurting. They are also approachable and willing to accept feedback even when it disagrees with their viewpoint.

For the past ten years, Jo has been an administrative assistant in a hospital. Most of the time, she works behind the scenes, managing program information for the medical records department.

But whenever there is a department meeting that involves critical decisions, the staff turns to Jo and asks for her input. Staff members know that Jo has the background and knowledge to advise the group on feasibility of new programs or changes to existing ones. Even though Jo doesn't have a title or employees who report to her, she demonstrates great leadership.

I have found some of the strongest and most compassionate leaders in similar positions. In my consulting work with churches, schools and hospitals, I usually start by having conversations with the administrative and support staff.

The cost of poor leadership

One of the staff members at a large organization recently described the challenges of poor leadership. Because of a demanding manager in one work area, several employees had transferred to another department and two other workers had resigned. Within a month, the company's clients were leaving, and sales were plummeting.

Since there wasn't a valid reason to fire the problem manager, the company leaders decided to wait it out and see if things improved. But they actually got worse, and employees in that department filed a complaint with human resources about the way they were being treated by the bad manager.

Finally, the owners stepped in and took action. First they transferred the problem manager to a different department in the company. Then they hired Les to become the new director for the problem area.

On his first day, Les set up a schedule for visiting all of the thirty employees who reported to him. With each one, he sat down in that person's cubicle or office and asked them what was going well and what needed work. Then he assured the staff members that he would address the problems quickly and invited them to stop in to visit any time they needed to talk.

A week later, he took all of the administrative staff to lunch and asked them about what they believed would improve the department. He also formed a small committee that gave him critical feedback on decisions made by higher management.

Les exuded compassion for those he worked with, and over time, clients returned and sales began to climb. Because of his caring style, his employees worked harder and helped him achieve the best sales results the department had seen in years. In this company, showing compassion for staff had a huge effect on the organization's bottom line.

Showing compassion at work

You may already strive to be a compassionate leader. But what about times when you have challenging employees or disagreements among your team members? I'm not going to teach you how to be a great boss or deal with employee issues. Instead, I want to give you a few key ways to show compassion to all of your employees and co-workers.

Let go of judgment

Instead of assuming someone is lazy or unmotivated, take time to build a connection with that person. Remember, you don't know the whole story.

Listen longer

The first thing a worker complains about is usually not the real problem. Listen longer and encourage dialogue. You may discover concerns or struggles you didn't even know about.

Appreciate everyone

Whenever possible, offer kind words and praise within earshot of a boss or supervisor. With time, you will become known as someone who notices and appreciates those around you.

Former President Jimmy Carter, known for a lifetime of service with Habitat for Humanity, encourages people to always be compassionate leaders. He said, "I have one life and one chance to make it count for something." He continued by affirming, "My faith demands that I do whatever I can, wherever I am, whenever I can, for as long as I can with whatever I have, to try to make a difference."

CHAPTER 13

Compassion in Churches

AS YOU KNOW, my wife is a breast cancer survivor. She went through major surgery, but her cancer was early stage so she didn't need to have chemotherapy or radiation. However, the early months of recovery were extremely hard for her. She was put on a medication that gave her lots of side effects as well as making her anxious and discouraged.

At that time, we were attending a church that had a special custom in its Sunday morning services. During the prayer time, worshippers were invited to come to the front of the church and kneel at the communion rail to pray. As they felt led to, some of the church members would join those at the rail, put hands on people's shoulders and pray for their needs.

One Sunday when my wife was having an especially hard time, she went forward, knelt at the rail and started to cry. Within a minute, she felt many hands on her shoulders and heard the quiet voices of those who joined her, asking God for comfort and help with whatever she needed that day.

With the compassion of those kind church members, that moment became a turning point in my wife's recovery. Soon after that, she started on a different medication that made her life a lot easier.

My wife and I celebrate that she has been a successful breast cancer survivor for many years. She still remembers the power and encouragement of receiving compassion when she needed it most.

Compassionate churches

If there is anywhere we would expect to see compassion shown and expressed, it's in the church community. The good news is that in the theology of most churches, compassion is central. By promoting healing, acceptance, support and connection, a church can become an oasis for those who enter its doors.

Unfortunately, over the past decades, church attendance has fallen considerably. This has made it harder for congregations to stay connected with regular attendees or to welcome visitors. In many churches, it's challenging for members to notice the needs around them and demonstrate compassion on a regular basis.

One of the ways churches can change this pattern is to create an identity of being a *compassionate church*. To do this, churches have to be intentional about showing kindness and caring for everyone who enters their doors.

Olivia Graham, a British bishop with the Church of England, has proclaimed that all churches should strive to be compassionate institutions. Here's how she describes a compassionate church:

> *A church should be a community of those who love and enfold the lonely, the sad, the grieving, the sick and the desperate. Members should strive to show warmth, understanding and acceptance.*
>
> *A compassionate church speaks in voices that welcome the stranger, the outsider, and the one who is different. This church knows that its fellowship will be enriched when these individuals become friends.*

In my own ministry, I've seen many wonderful examples of compassionate churches. They tend to provide a community people want to belong to, value people by remembering them and calling them by name, and respond with caring to stories of pain and suffering.

I've also attended a new style of church that focuses on providing a great worship experience but doesn't offer classes or programs. The services tend to be entertaining and often very meaningful. But it's easy to walk into the building, participate in the service, and then go home without speaking to anyone.

These churches might get strong attendance but don't make it easy to receive compassion during times when you need it. For me personally, I want to feel welcomed and cared about when I attend church. I also want a place where I can build friendships and connections.

A place to belong

For many years, the television sitcom *Cheers* depicted an environment where the people were glad to see each other and offered support for daily challenges. They laughed together, cried together, and were always aware when someone was missing.

The show's theme song declared the little tavern would always be a place "where everybody knows your name." They demonstrated compassion in their relationships, forgiving when someone made a mistake and offering encouragement when someone struggled or feared tomorrow.

Most of us yearn to have places where we belong. Whether it's family, a sports team or an organization, we want to be recognized and greeted by people who "know our name." Churches have a unique opportunity to accomplish this.

Because of my background as a minister and chaplain, I tend to have high expectations for a church home. My wife and I have visited many churches and have seen some great examples of feeling welcomed as well as a few places that left us feeling alone and disappointed.

It starts with "hello"

When you first enter the doors of a new church, you want someone to notice you and help you feel comfortable. Many churches have team members who greet regular attendees but also try to recognize visitors and give them extra attention. Of course, this depends on the size of the congregation, but for smaller churches, it's not that hard to do.

At one of our churches, greeters welcomed people by saying, "Good morning. We are glad you are here." Once they knew someone was visiting, they would add, "Can I be of help in any way? I can show you where to hang your coat, find the nursery, or locate a Sunday School classroom."

At one megachurch where it's easy to get lost, the greeters stand in the middle of the church entry and make an effort to notice anyone who seems new or is looking for directions. They also wear bright green shirts that say, "Can I be of help?"

Sometimes I've had greeters say, "Please remind me of your name." That showed they remembered me and it made me feel welcomed. Another greeter told me, "I'm usually standing by this tall counter in the entryway. I'll watch for you next week."

Many churches provide visitors with a "welcome gift" that contains information about their ministries. But one of my favorite ones came from a greeter who said, "Here is a welcome packet and it contains three coupons for free drinks in our coffee shop."

At another church, a greeter walked my wife and me toward the sanctuary and said to an usher, "We have new friends here today. Please help them find a comfortable place to sit."

Instead of immediately showing us to seats, the usher asked us if we had a preference on where we'd like to sit. She also asked whether we needed to be close to the front so we could hear the service better. Then she guided us toward a row about halfway from the back which fit our needs perfectly.

Once when we attended a very large church, we looked for visitor parking and easily found a spot fairly close to the door. A parking attendant immediately headed our way and said he was glad to see us and he hoped we would enjoy the service.

When we returned to our car, there was a large green card tucked under our windshield wiper that said, "We are so happy you joined us today. Let us know how we can help you in your faith journey. Here's how to reach us…" and it gave the phone number for the main office.

If the church size allows it, I recommend that all the adults wear name tags. Even if many of the church members know each other, name tags help visitors feel comfortable asking questions about the church and its ministries. It also helps people avoid feeling embarrassed about not remembering someone's name.

Are you alone?

We tend to care for people who look like us, share similar backgrounds, or are in the same age group. But sometimes we need to watch for the people who appear left out or alone.

One congregation designated a couple staff members each Sunday to watch for people who were sitting by themselves. They would approach these individuals and say, "It looks like you don't have anyone else here. May I sit with you?" This simple invitation was usually well received and even remembered later by visitors who felt welcomed and cared about.

Sal was an older gentleman whose care center took him to church each week. Once he arrived, Sal was usually led to a place at the end of a row where he readied himself for worship. When it came time for communion, the people in front of Sal filed out, but he didn't move.

One Sunday, Janet, a woman who was sitting several rows behind him, noticed Sal sitting and waiting. She quietly edged up the rows and asked Sal if he would like to go up to communion with her. He said, "Yes. That would be wonderful."

Janet took his arm and they headed to the communion rail at the front of the church. After the service that day, she learned that Sal was nearly blind, and he appreciated her compassionate act of helping him to communion. From that point on, she made sure that someone was always available to walk Sal to the communion rail.

Changing times

Church potlucks and women's circles used to provide ways to connect and visit. They also helped people learn about church members who were ill or struggling and made it easy to visit the sick or bring meals after an illness or a death.

But with the drop in church attendance, groups such as women's ministries struggle to stay active and significant. Unfortunately, the need to be with people who know us and care about our life struggles hasn't gone away.

Some church leaders gather a team of volunteers who visit ill church members and shut-ins as well as deliver meals or offer rides to medical appointments. One church we know of uses an online program called Meal Train to organize meal delivery for members who had surgery.

Another church has a hospitality ministry called "Make, Bake and Take." This group provides meals that are mostly casseroles or main dishes that can be frozen and used as needed. People who received these meals were extremely grateful for having food for their families without having to plan, shop and cook.

A couple years ago, in a nearby town, a family's son was murdered. During the murder trial, the victim's family members stayed at the courthouse every day to watch the proceedings and support each other. Unfortunately, if they left the courthouse, they were not allowed to return until the next day. That meant no lunch breaks or ways to bring in food.

Once their church members learned about this, they worked on a plan to help the family. For 14 days, they brought lunch to the courthouse and dropped it off for all of the family members. In this unusual act of compassion, the church made a significant difference helping this family cope during such a painful time.

Compassion through small groups

In recent years, small groups have become popular in churches and are providing new ways to connect. The model varies, but many of the groups meet in homes where members share coffee or meals, do Bible studies and pray for each other. When someone is ill or has surgery, group members learn about it quickly and can provide meals or visits.

While small groups provide an excellent ministry, they are not a good option for everyone. Matching people with other group members requires careful planning and support.

Churches also need to have ways for people to learn about groups and try them out without being pressured to join one. At one of the churches we attended, all of the small groups were posted on a large bulletin board in the lobby. Each listing had a photo of the leaders and described the age brackets and interests of that specific group. We noticed that many of the groups had a note saying, "Group is full but we will make room for you."

Somehow that simple line showed compassion and made us feel welcomed and wanted. It also gave us courage to contact the leaders of groups we were interested in, and we were able to find a group that matched our needs.

If you have a small-group ministry at your church, be sure to consider ways to accommodate people who don't fit the model. For example, evening groups might not be right for older people who don't want to drive at night or for those who live a distance from the meeting location.

One church has a Sunday School class that has met as a small group for years. Each week, the class begins with a discussion question that helps people feel connected. For example, leaders might ask, "What did you do for the recent holiday?" or "Did you have pets when you were growing up?"

The goal is to ask something that is personal but safe to talk about. Everyone takes a turn answering the question and sometimes the class members laugh and talk so much they hardly have time for the Bible lesson.

At the end of class each week, the leaders pass around a "Prayer sheet" and anyone who wants to can share prayer requests or personal needs. The prayer sheet is then scanned and emailed to everyone in the group. The next week, the class members report answers to prayer or updates to health or personal concerns. This model has built great depth in the relationships, and the participants have done many acts of caring and compassion for each other.

Two by Four friendship program

One of our churches regularly offers women's lunches and presentations which are well attended. But when we surveyed the church women, we learned that most who attended those events enjoyed visiting with people at their lunch tables, but found it hard to stay connected or build friendships with each other.

Based on creative ideas from a few women, we started a program called "Two by Four." The first month, each woman was paired with another person, which made the "two." Once they received the names and contact information of their assigned partners, each group of two would set up a time and place to meet.

The following month, each group of two was paired with two more women, which made the "four," and they would plan a meeting. We encouraged the pairs and groups to meet in person for coffee, lunch or even a walk. If an in-person meeting was difficult, they could also connect by phone, email or even text.

At each of the meetings, the participants took turns introducing themselves and sharing things about where they grew up, their home or work, family situation, children and other details. We often provided a conversation starter question that helped them begin their discussions.

Next, they talked about what was going on in their lives, sharing good things as well as challenges. At the end of the meetings, the participants asked each other, "What can I pray about for you?" and together they agreed to include those needs in daily prayers.

They were also encouraged to stay in touch with their partners and update them on life changes or answers to prayers. The church women loved the Two by Four program, and many of them built new friendships that have lasted for years.

We offered this program three times a year, and each term lasted two months. Those who wanted to participate could sign up for all three terms or for only the ones that matched their schedules.

Because of rotating the partners and groups each time, it takes a bit of organizing to make this work. But we found using a computer spreadsheet made it easy to track the progress and change the partner assignments each term.

In addition to the church, my wife also used the Two by Four program with a local women's group here in Iowa. Instead of asking about prayer requests, she simply changed the final question to "What gives you meaning, makes you happy or brings you joy in life?" The group members built many new friendships as a result of the program.

Compassion through prayer

During my ministry years, I often visited church members who were ill or not able to leave their homes. During these visits, I always read a few Scripture verses to the people and then prayed with them. I loved being able to use prayer as a way to show my compassion for these individuals.

But there have been many times in our lives when my wife and I were the ones needing compassion. I will always be grateful for the people who cared about us and offered to pray for our needs.

When I was ready to retire from my teaching job, we decided to move from Colorado to Iowa, where my wife's family lived. Unfortunately, we put our house up for sale during a time when the market was really slow. After trying for six months to get a buyer, we felt discouraged as well as worried about the impending time crunch for our move.

At our church, everyone was asked to complete a weekly "attendance card" that showed who was there each Sunday. Usually we just wrote our names and dropped the card in the offering plate. But one day, we turned the card over to the area where we could list prayer requests. We wrote a simple note about the need to get our home sold quickly since we were getting close to our moving date. Then we slid the card into the offering plate as usual. Two weeks later we had a buyer for our house.

The following Sunday, we were visiting with people in the entryway of the church, and an elderly lady stopped us and asked, "Are you Mike and Linda Spangle?" We told her yes and asked why. She immediately said, "I wondered if you've had any luck with selling your house."

Then she explained, "I am part of the prayer committee and you were on my personal list of people to pray for. Since I got your request a couple weeks ago, I have been praying for you every single day."

We had tears in our eyes as we told her about the answer to her prayers. Her heart for us felt amazing and reminded us that prayers are always a way to show compassion.

Tell me!

Sometimes people who might go unnoticed demonstrate some of the best examples of compassion. They are the quiet church members who become encouraging and supportive prayer warriors.

At one church, a grandmother regularly welcomed people to her home for visits. When people were struggling with life challenges or wanting help with decisions, they knew Grandma would be ready to help. She never talked much, but each time, she listened for as long as people needed.

The routine was always the same. People would call and ask if they could come over. Once they arrived, Grandma would make tea. After she filled the tea cups, she would sit down and demand, "Tell me!"

That simple invitation resulted in many hours of talking, sharing and sometimes crying. When the time was right, Grandma finished the meetings by saying, "I invite you to pray with me. Is that OK?"

Then she would put all of the concerns into a heartfelt prayer that made it feel as if God was there in the room, listening and guiding lives. For many years, Grandma's compassion brought comfort and healing to those who were blessed to know her.

CHAPTER 14
Compassion and Forgiveness

ONE OF THE SADDEST THINGS in my work is hearing someone say, "I'll never forgive them for what they did!" This statement typically comes from people who are struggling with relationships, usually family members or friends.

Unfortunately, being unwilling to forgive can prevent these people from finding peace and happiness in their lives. It can also get in the way of moving forward with important challenges, including financial decisions.

Some years ago, two sisters asked me to help them negotiate with their brother George about a family issue. Their father had died recently, and in his will, he left a high-rise apartment building to George and his sisters. However, the will stipulated the siblings all had to agree on the terms of the sale.

Several potential buyers had made offers to purchase the building, but George would always reject them based on small, insignificant issues. After many unsuccessful attempts to reach a compromise, the family decided to meet with a lawyer. In an initial, private conversation with the attorney, George said, "I won't agree to anything until they resolve the issue of the glove."

Then George explained that when he was about 8 years old, he was on the way to school when his sisters took his wool glove and played keep-away from him in the snow. They laughed and teased and made fun of him, even called him a sissy. He said, "I will never forget that humiliating day, and until they apologize, I won't agree to the terms of the building sale."

When the attorney and I met with the family, we asked the sisters if they were ready to resolve the issue about the glove. They both laughed, and then one of them said, "That is ridiculous! He was such a sissy when he was little, and he still is. He just has to get over it."

But without receiving an apology, George left the meeting and refused to approve the sale of the building. Because the sisters were unwilling to show compassion, the sale fell through, and over the next many years, this situation cost the family a lot of money. I don't know if they ever reached an agreement about selling the building.

Forgiveness and compassion

I've thought about that glove many times over the years. In my work, I have seen a lot of families who are unwilling to express forgiveness for emotional pain they've caused each other. I always feel sad when I see people refuse to forgive and I watch their relationships crumble.

George wanted his sisters to "pay" for doing harm, and he refused to let go of his anger and resentment. That's like holding a hot coal in your hand as you "show them" they can't treat you that way. But who is getting burned by that hot coal? It's certainly not the one you want to get even with.

Anger protects us in the moment of harm, but as time goes by, it outlives its usefulness. Eventually anger prevents us from living with emotional freedom. Instead of focusing on what went wrong, we need to shift our thinking to how good it feels to let go of negative emotions that no longer serve any useful purpose.

One of my students held anger for years about losing his girlfriend to one of his friends. During our class on forgiveness, he told me, "I thought my anger was hurting him. Then I discovered it was only hurting me. They both went on with their lives, and now it's time for me to get on with mine."

When forgiveness happens, compassion can come forward. And while it can't undo the past, nurturing memories that are touched by compassion can repair a lot of emotional harm. This doesn't mean we need to forget the past. It simply means we need to focus on examples of compassion in our past and use that to heal our relationships.

If George had reflected on some of the good times in his childhood, he might have pulled up compassionate memories instead of angry, judgmental ones. He also didn't realize that as long as he stayed angry at people, they controlled his life. It looked to me like George's stubbornness kept him from feeling peaceful and happy.

Memories may not be correct

Research shows that when we are emotionally harmed, our brain sends out a series of messages. It might tell us our pride has been wounded. Or it might suggest that others don't like us or that someone is a bad person. It also tells us that in order to protect ourselves, we must never forget what has happened.

However, psychologists have found that vivid memories about distressful events are often not accurate. We tend to remember how we felt at the time, but forget some of the details that caused the problem. We may have even said or done something that triggered the harm, but our mind chooses to block those memories.

Sally's 11-year-old daughter was exceptionally good at swimming, and she began competing in swim meets at her school. Sally's mom asked if she could come and watch the meets, but Sally refused. She still held a lot of grudges toward her mother because of things that had happened in her own childhood. But her mom persisted in requesting to come and watch her granddaughter's swim meets.

Finally Sally asked me to visit with her and her mother to figure out how they could get along better. In our meeting, Sally told how her mother had never attended her school contests and events. Because Sally's father had left them many years before, she felt alone and abandoned during those times.

Her mother listened quietly, then said, "Most of the time during your early school years, I was working two jobs to provide a home and food for us. I am so sorry that my work kept me from being there when you needed me."

Sally was shocked! As a young child, she hadn't realized how hard her mother had worked to take care of them. Her childhood memories focused on only her own feelings, not her mom's struggle to make a decent living. With tears on her face, she hugged her mother and said she was sorry for holding a grudge all those years. She also invited her mom to start coming to the swim meets, starting that afternoon.

Replacing anger

Psychologist and forgiveness specialist Everett Worthington teaches a concept called "emotional replacement." He encourages us to replace emotions of anger or hate with feelings that are more constructive. For example, instead of anger, we might recognize our disappointment in how another person behaved. Or we might say that we are sad or discouraged about a broken relationship.

The next time you feel angry, write the words, "I'm angry and I'm also..." on a piece of paper. Then make a list of other words such as disappointed, hurt, sad or frustrated. By identifying emotions besides anger, you'll get a more accurate picture of the situation and why it upset you. Once you weaken your anger feelings, you might be able to forgive the person who made you angry.

Worthington says, "You can whack away at unforgiveness with a giant dose of empathy, sympathy, compassion or love, and simply overwhelm it." He characterizes this as a "love bomb" that blows the bad feelings to bits and allows you to forgive the wrongs.

What's the real issue?

When Tom started a new job, a co-worker welcomed him but confided that she had wanted the job he had gotten. Then she insisted that he check with her before making any major decisions. Tom wasn't sure about this and basically ignored her request. Over the next year, this co-worker made Tom's life so difficult that he decided to leave the company.

At first, he was angry and resentful about what this co-worker had done. He told me, "I can't imagine forgiving her and showing her kindness when I see her again." But eventually Tom heard from others that she had been passed over for promotions several times. She had few friends and didn't appear to enjoy her work. It seemed that she needed to hurt others in order to stay confident in her own position.

Once he learned about her background, Tom began to understand why she had acted in such hurtful ways. At that point, he began to soften his view toward her and eventually moved past his anger with her.

Figuring out how to have empathy when you've been wronged can be a challenge. But as Tom did, you can start by trying to understand the situation and what prompted the harmful actions. Sometimes you see a lack of social skills or people's inability to filter what they say or do.

I have also seen times when people are so miserable in their own lives that they say or do things to make others miserable as well. Some people feel a sense of power in manipulating others or creating dramas that make them appear strong while others look bad.

Feeling empathy for someone who has harmed you doesn't mean you condone the actions. You also don't have to believe you deserved the harm or allow that person to harm you again. But you don't need to let harm ruin your life or steal your joy.

Writer and poet, Maya Angelou has a wonderful quote that reminds us, "You may not control all the events that happen to you, but you can decide not to be reduced by them." In other words, letting go of anger helps you move on from the events and seek happiness and peace.

Forgiving nothing

Compassionate empathy recognizes that sometimes we need to forgive someone's failures including the absence of actions. In other words, we may need to forgive others for doing nothing when we yearned for caring or love.

A 30-year-old student came to see me because she was struggling with her classes. She was drinking and partying a lot and knew she was risking her education as well as other areas in her life. She blamed her father for all of this.

When I asked what he did that was so awful, she answered, "Nothing. It's what he didn't do. He was a farmer and I know he was usually tired at the end of the day. But he seemed to forget I existed.

"If I came home from school with good grades, he would glance at my report card and grunt. I wanted him to tell me that he was proud of me and that he was amazed I could do so well in school.

"When I was in high school, my parents left for a weekend and I took care of the farm while they were gone. I milked the cows, ran the cream separator, gathered eggs, and fed all the animals. It was a challenge because I was also doing homework and studying for tests.

"After they got home, I waited for my father to show how much he appreciated what I had done. He asked if everything went OK, but then walked away and never even thanked me for my work. I still hold a lot of anger toward him for never showing me love or attention."

Over several meetings, the student and I talked about her home life and what was missing. She acknowledged that her father never physically harmed her or her siblings. He just stayed quiet about everything they did, good or bad.

Finally I asked her, "What if you accepted your father for the person he appears to be, not the person you wished he was? In other words, could you forgive him for being who he is?"

She spent the next week considering this unusual way to resolve her anger and resentment about her father. The next time we met, she tearfully said, "Yes, I have decided to do what you suggested. I will forgive him for what he didn't do. I will accept him for being who he is and begin to show him love instead of disappointment and frustration."

A month later, the student stopped in to see me and described a wonderful visit home where she hugged her father and thanked him for being there. He seemed surprised, but accepted her affection and told her he was glad she was happy. When she realized she couldn't change her father, she decided that forgiving him would resolve her anger and help her live a healthier life.

The connection

Compassion and forgiveness move both directions. Without forgiveness, it's hard to show empathy and caring. But at the same time, showing compassion becomes a doorway to forgiveness. It allows you to view life events from a perspective that gives you the courage to forgive. Sometimes we learn these principles through very painful events in life.

Mary was a schoolteacher who lived in Pennsylvania near an area with several Amish communities. One rainy evening at dusk, Mary was driving home on a narrow, two-lane road when an Amish farmer's horse and buggy pulled out in front of her.

She attempted to avoid the buggy, but unfortunately, she hit it hard enough to send it into the ditch. The accident killed the husband and wife who were in the front of the buggy but left alive a teenage daughter in the backseat.

As you would expect, Mary was devastated. Even though the police decided she was not at fault, Mary held herself accountable for the accident. For weeks she couldn't sleep and found herself crying every day.

Eventually Mary went to the small Amish town to visit the relatives of the family and express her sadness. Amazingly, she was met with open arms and a readiness to forgive. One elder said, "It must be God's will that these friends died and that their daughter lived."

It took a long time for Mary to move past the pain of the accident. But the tremendous compassion shown by the Amish family helped her heal as well as forgive herself. Since that time, Mary has become a deaconess in her church, and she teaches others how to forgive and show compassion, especially during times of tragedy.

Phases of forgiveness

Taking a compassionate approach toward forgiveness requires letting go of past thoughts about events and relationships. It also requires giving yourself permission to forgive. To do this, you have to release your negative feelings and decide that it's time to heal and get on with your life.

Forgiving others involves several phases or actions. The first one is telling yourself that you won't take any further actions toward the one who harmed you. Instead, you confirm that *all* is forgiven and you are not going to hold on to your anger any longer.

The second phase may take a while. It requires getting over lingering emotions that pop up or return, even though you have made the decision to forgive. You might enlist the help of a pastor or therapist to help you move through this phase.

But you also need to consciously remind yourself to let go of the past, including the bad feelings. Remember the concept of "emotional replacement" and start substituting thoughts of compassion and caring toward those who harmed you, even if they are no longer living.

The third phase involves moving past a bad experience sufficiently that you rarely think about it any more. This isn't an easy step because our brains want us to remember the details and replay them over and over. But with time, you can train yourself to let go of the painful thoughts and memories.

Freedom from old, unwanted thoughts involves viewing the past with compassionate forgiveness instead of judgment. Give your mind permission to focus on what is positive *now* instead of getting stuck in the past.

Let grace wash over all of your negative memories. Then allow your mind, perhaps through prayer or meditation, to develop new mental pathways that enable you to live the best life you can. Again, this does not diminish harms from the past. But it will help you live a full and beautiful life instead of one burdened by bitterness or resentment. It will also allow you to get back power and control in your life instead of having those things owned by others.

A good friend who went through some extremely painful and devastating events in his life said it this way:

I forgive because it makes me whole and healthier. It allows me to show compassion to everyone who comes across my path. And that's how I want to go through life.

CHAPTER 15

Barriers to Compassion

MANY DAYS you want to show compassion to people, but you can't seem to do it very well. Instead, you yell at other drivers or snap at people in your home. You don't mean to be impatient or unkind, but sometimes, you just don't feel very compassionate.

It's easy to understand why this happens. Fatigue, stress, or simply your busy life can all get in the way of showing compassion. But sometimes the cause goes deeper than those typical reasons.

A negative outlook on life or even old childhood messages can affect your ability to care about pain and suffering. Recognizing your barriers becomes the first step in moving past them and becoming a more compassionate person.

Childhood messages

When Sam was growing up, his home life was awful. His father was an alcoholic who yelled a lot when he'd been drinking. He constantly criticized Sam and his brothers and generally made their lives miserable.

On the day he turned 16, Sam left home, got a job and moved in with friends. When he and I talked about compassion, Sam told me, "I know that compassion is important in life, but because of my dad, I don't know what it looks like or how to show it."

Sam was great at his work as an engineer, but he struggled to get along with the other employees. He was fearful of being harmed, even by his work friends. He said, "It's hard for me to know who to trust. So I protect myself by staying quiet and working alone."

Even after many years, childhood messages can still influence your ability to show compassion. Your memories from the past overshadow your ability to care in the present. But if you look closely at those events, you might understand how your struggles to show compassion are not your fault.

Sam realized that 40 years later, he was still holding anger and resentment toward his father. It took some time, but he decided to stop letting his childhood get in the way of his life as an adult. Once he quit blaming his father for his current struggles, Sam was able to soften his view and show more caring toward others.

Isn't it awful!

In today's world, the daily news, television programs and social media all tell us what's going wrong. But rarely do these sources provide solutions to the problems. As a result, many people develop a negative mindset that gets in the way of being kind to others.

Neuroscience warns that our brains are drawn toward negative information more than toward positive events. So when media outlets show dramatic footage of hurricanes, protests or physical attacks, we become glued to the screen. But unless we protect our mental status, we can become infected with a negative global outlook.

We also know that negativity is contagious. So if you spend a lot of time around grouchy or pessimistic people, you'll begin to share their viewpoint. It's hard to show compassion to others when you feel cynical about the world around you.

To avoid sliding into a negative viewpoint, you have to intentionally change your thinking. For example, if you are with someone who has a litany of things wrong in life, ask that person to tell you about something that's going well. That may not stop a conversation completely, but at least you'll be able to see if that individual is harming your outlook.

In your own life, practice focusing on things that are positive and happy. Take time to notice the sunshine and the small surprises that brighten your day. An unexpected hug or a thank-you from someone can create a positive moment. In return, speaking kindly or greeting someone warmly will add to your own level of optimism.

Compassion grows in a positive climate. By focusing on what's positive, you can improve your emotional outlook on life as well as your ability to show compassion to others.

It's too big

When employees in a large manufacturing company go on strike, my first thought is, "I hope they get it settled." If I read about a business laying off a lot of workers, I think, "I hope those people find new employment."

But when I visited John, my next-door neighbor who had lost his job, I got a different view of the pain these people endure. John described the awful feelings of packing everything in his office into a couple of boxes, then being escorted out the door by security personnel.

Since then, he has lost touch with most of his colleagues, and he no longer has work friends who invite him out to lunch. Beside those losses and disappointments, John told me he doesn't know how he is going to pay his rent next month or buy school clothes for his children.

Suddenly the decisions of a big company came close to my home, and I immediately began feeling empathy for John and his family members. I decided to show compassion and I began helping him with some house projects. My wife and I watched John's kids so he could go job hunting. We brought meals to his home and gave him gift cards for groceries.

It might seem like the events at a company or business are thousands of miles away. But even those problems need our attention. To show compassion, you need to bring your empathy down to a level where you have some power.

When my brother-in-law travels with a disaster team, he knows they can't fix an entire town. But they show compassion at each home they work on, and their kindness matters to those who live there.

Workers at food pantries don't make a dent in world hunger. But as they watch grateful families leave with food for the next week's meals, they know their compassion has made a difference.

Every December one of my family members volunteers to ring a bell for Salvation Army fundraising. She can't readily help people who have experienced disasters. But she uses her volunteer work to show compassion for those who've been through a house fire or natural disaster.

She told me, "As I stand outdoors, ringing the bell in the cold and wind, I picture the families who are devastated by life events. And I keep ringing because it's a way I can show them compassion."

You don't know what it's like

With most of the suffering in our world, I don't have a clue what it's like for the people who are going through hard times.

As a kid, I complained about meals, but I never went to school hungry. I've never had my house burn down or lost all of my belongings in a flood.

Even though I can't understand what those things feel like, I can still respect loss and the challenges these people endure. I can seek to learn about people's pain and what they are feeling and needing right now.

The first step requires patiently listening and expressing concern for the person who is suffering. As you hear more of the story, empathy begins to stir, and eventually you might see a place or situation where you can offer help.

When talking with people going through hard times, I've learned ways to improve my knowledge and ability to show compassion. Here are some responses I might use:

- Help me understand what you are going through.
- Tell me what it feels like for you right now.
- Help me learn more about your life and your experiences.

Giving solutions instead of compassion

Too often we hear about someone's suffering or hardships and our first thought is, "They should..." followed by what we think is a great solution. But we are usually wrong. What looks simple is typically more complex.

For example, finding adequate child care is hard for most working parents. But it's even more challenging for a single mom or divorced parents who share custody but live far apart.

With aging parents, well-meaning adults explore assisted living or nursing home options. But sometimes their good intentions are blocked by the older adults who are not ready to leave the home they've lived in for decades.

As you listen to people describe their challenges, resist the temptation to offer advice or solutions. Instead, the best way to show compassion to these hurting individuals is patiently listening and nodding your head a lot. Catch yourself when you start saying, "You should..." because true compassion is not giving solutions.

I don't know what to say

We've all had it happen. We hear about a tragedy such as the death of a loved one, and we don't have a clue what to say or do. We try to be kind and utter the words, "I'm so sorry," but then we can't figure out what to do next. Since we don't know what to say, we try to offer comfort with lots of words.

But usually the person who's had the loss doesn't want to hear about what your uncle or grandmother went through when a family member died. Instead, someone who has lost a child or a life partner simply wants you to show compassion.

I recently interviewed a grief counselor and asked for help on how to show compassion after someone has experienced a great loss. The first thing I learned is to stop talking so much. Instead, I need to trust that my presence alone can be helpful to a grieving person. The counselor reminded me, "The greater the pain, the fewer the words should be said."

When you visit people who are grieving, it's always fine to start by saying, "I'm sorry." You can add, "I'm so sorry for your loss," and acknowledge how painful this must be for them. But after that, go silent. Sit with them and just be present for a few minutes. Even though it's painful to wait for people to respond, do it anyway.

Once they begin to speak, quietly listen to what they say. After a person has opened the conversation, you can offer kind words without saying a lot. Here are a few ideas:

- Yes, it must be really hard for you.
- I can't imagine what this feels like for you.
- My heart is with you right now.

Resist the temptation to offer platitudes such as, "It was God's will." Also, don't suggest someone can "have another child" or "find a new partner." When my wife and I lost our babies after problem pregnancies, we hated it when people said, "You can always try again." We wanted people to simply acknowledge our pain and sadness.

Remember that grief doesn't stop after a funeral. Sometimes people suffer more after their family members and friends have gone home. If you live close enough to someone who is grieving a loss, offer to visit at intervals over the weeks and months ahead. Bring flowers to replace the ones that have wilted.

Send "I'm thinking about you" cards that let people know you haven't forgotten about them and their pain. When they are ready, invite them to lunch at a quiet restaurant. Or ask if they want to meet for coffee. Stay in touch and let people know you haven't forgotten what they've been through.

The grief counselor also told me that birthdays, anniversaries and holidays are some of the hardest times for people who've lost a spouse or partner. Since you can't say "Happy Birthday" to someone who has died, it's easy to stay silent on those days. But during the first year or two, those times are the most painful ones for the survivor.

The counselor suggested that you help a grieving person avoid going through those events alone. For example, instead of pretending birthdays and anniversaries are not important, invite that person to do a "memory celebration." Have a meal together and talk about best memories of those days in years past. While there will still be tears and sadness, the grieving person doesn't have to sit alone on those painful days.

Compassionate lens

Look around and view what you see through eyes of compassion. You may be surprised at the many opportunities to do a simple act that shows a caring heart. Instead of approaching a conflict with the belief that one of us is wrong and the other is right, look for common ground. Explore ways to be more inclusive and open-minded.

Rather than instantly forming opinions about others, remember that you don't know their story. Compassion requires letting go of rigid thinking and accepting there are many ways to think and behave. It also forces you to let go of judgments and assumptions about others. Instead, you have to open your heart to the possibility that others may not think or act the same way as you.

It's too close to home

Psychologist Paul Gilbert believes our ability to feel compassion is related to our "distress tolerance." He explains that the ways we manage our own emotions becomes harder when we encounter a similar problem in someone else.

If we over-identify with someone's suffering, we may struggle to feel compassion for that person. For example, listening to someone talk about marital problems may be uncomfortable if you've had similar relationship issues. If you haven't worked through your own feelings about a parent's death, it may be hard to express compassion for someone with a parent who is dying.

For most of our issues, the passage of time brings healing. Eventually, we might find we can be more empathetic about other people's struggles because of our own experiences. In some cases, going through suffering ourselves may be the best training for showing compassion to others.

Wise compassion

Displaying compassion for someone's distress will always involve some level of risk. I might fear my actions will be rejected. Or I might realize the situation requires a greater level of involvement or time than I am willing to give.

In his book *The Most Good You Can Do*, Peter Singer encourages us to approach acts of compassion with "effective altruism." That requires investing your efforts in a way that will do the greatest good. For example, referring my depressed student to a counselor who could provide lasting help was a stronger path than my limited words of encouragement.

Sending a financial gift to a group that feeds and clothes homeless people may be more effective than giving money to someone begging on a street corner. In other words, compassion should be linked to wisdom about how to best respond to a situation.

Of course, sometimes we are surprised with the outcome of acts of compassion. Many years ago, I took a group of high school students to a center for children with Down syndrome or other intellectual disabilities. I was nervous because these students would see children who were different than any they had encountered before.

There was the potential that the students would see only the negative aspects of these children and fail to show compassion. But that isn't what happened. With their innocent, outreached hands, the young Down syndrome children brought smiles to the students. It was clear they viewed us as welcome friends. In response, my students expressed compassion for the children and returned the smiles and hugs.

In the years that followed, many of these students continued their relationships with people who were emotionally or physically challenged. Several of my students regularly volunteered to help with the Special Olympics organization. They told me amazing stories about playing sports or being in the cheering section alongside these special individuals. My students also described how their efforts to show compassion helped them become stronger and more caring in all areas of their lives.

CHAPTER 16

Compassion Fatigue

IN THE EARLY YEARS of my career, I thought I could do it all. For a time, I served as an instructor at two different universities and pastored a small mission church 40 miles into the mountains outside of Denver. I also served as a part-time youth pastor for a city church and a part-time chaplain for the Navy Reserve.

I loved all of my roles, but some weeks, especially if there were weddings or funerals, I felt exhausted. Emotionally, I was involved in many lives with different and difficult kinds of problems. I didn't know how to say "no," and I had high expectations for myself in each of my roles.

At times, I felt as though I was going through the motions, and I knew I wasn't emotionally present with people. I began feeling doubt about my career, and I wondered if this was the work I should be doing.

Finally, I realized I had to make some hard decisions about where I wanted to invest my time and energy. I withdrew from the two church jobs and switched to teaching at only one school. I started playing tennis to get regular exercise. Within a couple months, I felt like a new person. My passion for helping people returned, and I began enjoying my work again.

We all can reach points in life where we have nothing left to give. And when you are the one who needs a hug or appreciation, it can be difficult to care about others.

During the years when my wife was working as a nurse, I saw many times when she became worn down and struggled with having compassion. Here's how she described one of those times.

I recognized it the minute it happened. I'd been on duty at my hospital nursing job for less than an hour when I found her again. An elderly female patient who was confused kept crawling over the rails of her bed in an effort to escape. Each time, I would untangle her limbs, get her positioned back into the bed and gently tuck in the pillows that kept her in place.

But the third time I entered her room and found her dangling precariously over the rails, I lost my patience. I quickly maneuvered her back into her bed, but when I looked down, I realized I was shaking her! At that exact moment, I knew I'd crossed the line from being a warm, caring nurse and entered the category of compassion fatigue. Linda S.

How does this happen?

I've heard many stories about loss of compassion from people in helping professions such as health and education. Social workers describe anxiety and guilt about feeling apathetic toward their work. Teachers speak of low energy, irritability and impatience with their students. Physicians talk about feeling less joy in their work or having struggles with exhaustion.

Janet, one of my work colleagues, had been feeling tired and not sleeping well for months. As a therapist in private practice, she kept pushing herself in spite of the fatigue. She told me, "If I don't see clients, I have no income. So I'm stuck, and I have to keep working."

But when she saw her doctor for the third time in a couple of months, he startled her by saying, "I'm firing you as a patient. I can't do anything more for you until you change your life pattern. You are taking care of everyone but yourself, and those people are *not* the ones sitting in my office right now."

Psychologists estimate that nearly 80 percent of helping professionals will experience compassion fatigue at some point in their careers. Workers describe feeling burned out or losing passion for work they used to love.

The constant demands of caring for others can wear people out, putting them at risk of developing compassion fatigue. It may show up as apathy, moodiness, sadness and in extreme cases, depression. Some people even become cynical or angry at the factors that contribute to their loss of compassion.

While people in helping professions are especially at risk of developing compassion fatigue, it can happen to anyone. People working in high-stress jobs can get worn down and lose passion for their work. The demands of children or the needs of aging parents can make people exhausted and impatient.

But people with the highest risk of compassion fatigue are those who are ongoing caregivers. Routinely taking care of a disabled child, someone with Alzheimer's disease or a person with a terminal illness can wear you down to a point of caregiver burnout. Even with someone you dearly love, you might wonder how much longer you can keep up with the person's demands and needs.

Signs of compassion fatigue

Sometimes compassion fatigue happens quickly and you suddenly lose your patience and yell at someone in frustration. But it can also creep into your life without you realizing it. At its worst, compassion fatigue can cause a mental breakdown that requires counseling or medical care.

The key to managing compassion fatigue is to recognize the signs before they take over your life. Here are some things to watch for:

- Decreased passion or joy in your work
- Becoming irritated, grouchy or impatient with people you are trying to help
- Feeling tired all the time, getting sick easily, not sleeping well
- Dreading going to work or meeting with clients
- Feeling depressed, lacking creativity or focus in your work
- Rarely getting a break from being a caregiver for a family member

The empty bucket

Most of the time, compassion fatigue doesn't happen overnight. It slowly creeps up on you over time, and it can be brought on by any number of events or actions. But most of the time, it shows up after you've given out huge amounts of compassion without taking care of your own spirit.

To understand the concept of emotional energy, picture a large container such as a water bucket. Inside this bucket, you have a constantly shifting level of positive emotional energy. When you are feeling healthy and balanced in your life, your bucket level will be at least half-full. Ideally, you start each day this way.

But just like physical energy, you have a limited amount of emotional energy. As you go through your day, demands from people, stress from your job or family, even the weather can take a toll on it. At the same time, positive things increase the emotional energy in your bucket. Kindness, affirmations, self-care and nurturing can all help move the level back up.

If you have lots of positive things in your life, your emotional energy climbs and life feels good. But during times when you deal with a lot of negatives or drainers, your emotional energy drops below the minimal level. By the end of the day, you are exhausted emotionally as well as physically.

If you don't refill your emotional bucket at intervals, you can reach a point where it's empty day after day. At some point, even the most caring, concerned individuals can slip into this crisis, and with it comes compassion fatigue.

Filling your emotional bucket

Recovering from compassion fatigue can take a long time. You might need an extended rest time or even a complete break from your life demands. In some cases, you can take a sabbatical from your job or arrange for someone to spend time with the people you care for.

But sometimes these breaks are not possible or practical. When that's true, you need to look for small steps that can give you a respite from your life challenges. For example, a friend whose husband has Alzheimer's disease was able to hire part-time caregivers who came to her home for a couple of afternoons each week.

During that time, my friend would meet people for lunch or go to a coffee shop on her own. She found that reading a favorite book and enjoying a quiet cup of coffee helped rebuild her emotional energy. After one of those afternoon breaks, she usually had far more patience and ability to take care of her husband's needs again.

To begin recovering from compassion fatigue, think about what fuels you and helps you feel more positive. Look for positive people who are energy builders instead of drainers. Draw on things that nurture you or increase your sense of meaning in life.

By taking care of your emotional bucket at intervals, you'll prevent it from getting so low that you feel drained and empty. Each day, plan a few things that will move your level of emotional energy back up, even just a little.

Sometimes it helps to think about what rejuvenated your spirit in the past. I love taking long walks in a nearby park that has a small lake in it. Even during my most challenging times, watching the movement of the water and listening to the birds in the nearby trees refuels me. I also love to sit in my big recliner chair and read for an hour. Even petting my dog or taking a warm bath helps me feel renewed.

I encourage you to create your own list of favorite things that help you refuel your spirit. Do those often and protect the times you set aside for them. By deepening your self-care, you'll find healing from emotional pain as well as compassion fatigue.

Focus your attention

Clinical psychologist Paul Gilbert provides insight on how to get your emotional life back on track when you experience compassion fatigue. He says, "Our attention functions like a spotlight—whatever it shines on becomes brighter in our mind."

The way we focus that spotlight affects us physically, emotionally and spiritually. Often we are not aware of how much we are shining a spotlight on the negative things in life.

If you are feeling discouraged or worn down, pay attention to your mental images and where you are focusing your energy.

Dr. Gilbert suggests that to prevent getting caught in a negative spiral, we need to take control of our spotlight. He tells us to focus our attention on the positive people and events in our lives. At the same time, we can send the negative ones into darkness, far away from our attention spotlight.

In my work as a professor, at the end of each class, I receive a set of student evaluations. Typically there will be a lot of glowing, positive reviews about the class and my teaching. But often one or two evaluations will be quite negative or contain criticism of the class.

Because our brain's natural instinct causes us to focus on the negative, I might feel anxious or even angry about the students who complained. When I go home and review my day with my wife, I will talk a lot about the "bad" students who gave me negative feedback. In other words, I get obsessed with the negative reviews and forget about the positive ones.

It's taken some effort, but I have worked hard at changing that pattern. If I get a negative evaluation for a class, I glance at it quickly to see if there's helpful information in it. Then I push it away and focus my spotlight on the positive reviews. I might read those several times over a couple of days. That simple change takes away my anger and frustration over the few negative comments.

When you are struggling with compassion fatigue, look around for positive things to put into your spotlight. Perhaps the sun is shining, you're reading a great book, or your kids are having fun with a new game. Force yourself to notice lots of good things in your life.

As you focus your attention on happier things, you'll be able to push some of the difficult or sad ones away from your spotlight. Even a brief respite from the challenges of your situation can renew your spirit and help you continue to show caring and compassion.

Managing compassion fatigue

When your roles involve caring for the needs of others, think about the outcomes you want to see as a result of your compassion. Perhaps your goal is to provide comfort and safety to someone with Alzheimer's disease or dementia.

Maybe you hope to see healing and recovery in a medical patient. Sometimes, you might simply want to provide support and encouragement that helps someone deal with grief or loss.

We can't fix the sadness and pain in our world, but showing compassion can help ease the suffering. Our job is to do the best we can in each situation and, at the same time, protect our own hearts and spirits.

Pay attention to how you talk about your situation. The way you describe your stress affects your emotional response to it. If possible, debrief your day with someone, but don't repeat the problems again and again. Rehearsing the situation might feel helpful but this lasts only a short time. Instead, try to engage in constructive discussions with a focus on how to improve the situations.

Preventing and managing compassion fatigue requires finding a balance between caring for others and caring for ourselves. Even in the most difficult settings, I encourage you to look for ways to take a break now and then from your efforts.

Here are a few strategies that might help:

- Set priorities on your daily tasks. Decide which ones can be put aside, at least for the time being.
- Consider the activities that used to refill your emotional reserves. Perhaps you could put some of them back into your life.
- Identify trigger events that begin to drain your energy. See if there's a way to avoid those situations, even for an hour or two.
- Decide if the number of responsibilities you are taking on is realistic. Allow or encourage others to accept more of the things you've been handling.
- Reclaim the spiritual side of your life. Find a place for quiet time and personal reflection. Or, if appropriate for you, say some prayers.

Family caregivers

Because there are many books and online resources available on the subject of family caregiver fatigue, I have not included a discussion of this area. I encourage you to seek out programs and support systems that will match your needs and your situation.

One of the best places to find content as well as local resources is Family Caregiver Alliance. This California company's mission is to improve the quality of the life for family caregivers and the people who receive their care.

The company's website, www.caregiver.org, provides extensive listings of programs and resources for every level of family caretakers. The site includes separate pages for each U.S. state, allowing you to find support systems and resources specific to your local area.

CHAPTER 17

Compassion Renewal

ONE MORNING a few years ago, I woke up feeling tired, grouchy and mad at the entire world. My work day was filled with meetings and teaching classes, and I couldn't imagine how I could be kind to my students and colleagues. I didn't feel the slightest bit compassionate toward anyone, even my dog!

I'm usually an upbeat kind of person, so this wasn't like me at all. I didn't like the way I was feeling, and I certainly didn't want to stay that way.

Over a few cups of coffee, I tried to figure out what was bothering me and why I had lost my caring spirit. Finally, I took out a piece of paper and wrote a list of some of the recent events in my life.

The month before my younger sister had died from cancer, and I was grieving her loss. From a couple thousand miles away, I was struggling to sell her mobile home and settle her meager estate. My car had needed major work, so I had some unexpected bills. At the university where I worked, rumors were circulating about budget cuts and potential staff layoffs.

As I looked at my list, I began to understand why I was feeling so down and uncaring. My life circumstances had drained me emotionally and left me feeling empty and sad.

After one more cup of coffee, I decided my first step was to get back in control of my life. To do that, I had to make some changes in my schedule and start taking better care of myself. But first I had to get through my work day.

After I got into my car, I said a prayer and asked for help with moving past my grouchy attitude. Then I started thinking about things I was grateful for. The list came quickly—sunshine, good health, a loving wife, a decent job, a car that worked and a home to live in.

The longer I focused on gratitude, the better I felt. And by the time I walked into my office, I knew I could be the caring, compassionate person I wanted to be that day.

Why does it leave?

We all understand the importance of compassion, but sometimes we just don't have the ability to show it. What happens to our compassion? Why does it leave, and how can we get it back?

As you know, compassion fatigue can occur when you've had to show kindness and caring for a long time. Health professionals and independent caregivers are always at risk for this. But stress, fatigue and real-life problems can affect any of us and cause us to lose the ability to show compassion.

Here are some of the most common reasons for losing our compassion:

- Grief and loss
- Relationship struggles
- Depression, anger, disappointment
- Feeling exhausted, worn out
- High levels of stress
- Fears about health, finances or other people

In my work, I've talked with many people who've struggled with their loss of compassion. Yet all of them desperately wanted to return to being a kind and caring person.

When I asked a group of physicians what prevented them from being more compassionate, one told me, "I love my work but often I become a victim of my schedule. It's hard to be compassionate when too many activities, even if they are worthwhile, have control over my life. Many times my only goal is getting through my day."

Steps to renewal

How can you recapture your joy and compassion in life when you are exhausted and worn down? A long vacation might seem like the best solution, but that's rarely possible at the time you need it most. Instead of dreaming of "someday" when you'll be able to slow down and take care of yourself, look for small ways to do self-care now.

On an airplane, you'll typically hear, "In case of a cabin pressure emergency, put your own mask on first before assisting others." This also applies to our daily lives. You can't help others for very long if you don't take care of yourself first.

Some things for self-care are easy. For example, healthy activities such as eating well and getting exercise will make you feel better. You also might want to work on rebuilding your confidence and self-esteem.

But here's a simple one. Get dressed every day, even if you don't think you'll see another person. Spending the day in pajamas or sweatpants won't improve your outlook on life, and that's an essential part of reviving your compassion. To heal your emotions and your caring heart, you need to demonstrate that you are strong and capable of self-care.

One of my favorite t-shirts has big letters saying, "NOPE. Not Today." I think all of us need more of that approach. Take a look at your daily life and consider whether you need to reset your priorities in order to get your life back in balance.

Ditch the negative

It's difficult to be a compassionate person if you are filled with negative thoughts. Anger and resentment crowd out the positive emotions that support a sense of well-being and give you the ability to care about others. If you're holding onto negative feelings or beliefs, it's time to work on letting them go.

Instead of assuming life can't get better, switch your view to believing that it *can*. Reframe the negative stories you tell yourself, and change the belief that something won't turn out right or that you can't be happy again. Instead, envision better endings for your stories, then work on making them come true.

Rethinking demands

During the years I was the pastor at a church in the mountains outside of Denver, I was asked to visit a family in crisis. I learned it was the second marriage for both parents and the new stepfather had high expectations and many rules for life in the home. The mother had become worried because arguments between the stepfather and her 15-year-old daughter were becoming louder and more dangerous.

When I sat down with the family, the parents described how the problems had escalated over the past year.

The stepfather began by complaining that the daughter came home late after school, had friends over while the parents were at work, and talked on the phone for hours every night. When the mother responded, she supported the role the stepfather took in setting down rules for the home.

The daughter tried to defend herself, but whenever she spoke, the stepfather interrupted. I noticed that as he pushed harder, the daughter pulled more into herself. I asked the parents to listen to her comments, but they were impatient, and whenever the daughter tried to speak, the parents kept talking at the same time.

After an hour, I suggested we resume the discussion in a few days after everyone had cooled down. However, the next morning, I got a distraught call from the stepfather telling me the daughter had run away. She left a note on her pillow that said, "I'm going away to find someone willing to listen to me." The parents had no idea where their daughter had gone, and they were unsuccessful in their attempts for find her.

Three years later, I heard from the daughter. She told me that she had gone to live with relatives several hundred miles away and that she was doing great. She was also inviting me to her wedding but mentioned that her mother and stepfather would not be attending. While I was happy for her, I felt sad and disappointed that her family members had lost so much connection in their lives together.

We rarely win hearts through louder arguments. Instead, we win them with understanding and negotiation. If these parents had looked for even small ways to show compassion, they might have prevented the situations that took their daughter away from them.

Focus on gratitude

Renewing your compassion begins with looking outward instead of inward. One of the simplest ways to do this is to practice gratitude or being thankful.

When you take time to appreciate what's good in your life, you shift your focus away from the challenges that drag you down. That doesn't take them away, but it helps you see past them and rediscover a spirit of caring.

One way to practice gratitude is to notice positive things that show up when you weren't even looking for them. Label these tiny bright spots as *rainbows*—gifts that slip in quietly, giving you an emotional boost right in the middle of an otherwise difficult day.

Look around you. Is the sun shining? Was someone kind to you at the bank or in the grocery store? Did you drink a great cup of tea this afternoon? While these may seem like small things, if you pay attention to your rainbows and appreciate them, they can totally change your outlook.

Noticing rainbows also involves being grateful for what's already there. For example, do you have at least one person who truly loves and accepts you? Did you recently finish reading an inspirational book or a great online article? Perhaps a song on the radio tugged at your emotions or brightened your spirit.

Cultivate a sense of gratitude about even the simple things that happen in your life. Be thankful each time your children arrive home safely after school. At bedtime, appreciate your cozy blanket and the way your pillow fluffs up under your head.

Consider keeping a gratitude journal. Write notes about your rainbows and consider all the ways they help you feel better. Let these small moments become opportunities for revitalizing your compassionate spirit.

Make it a habit to count your blessings. Choose a time each week to reflect on what is going well or what you are grateful for, then write these down. You might pick a specific number, such as three or five, and identify that many blessings each week.

Watch for places to feel joy. Don't put off feeling happy because you are waiting for things to improve! Instead, find pieces of joy in as many small life moments as possible.

During the first painful year after the death of her husband, a friend was determined not to lose sight of joy. She said, "Every morning when I get out of bed, I put my feet on the floor and tell myself that no matter how bad my grief is, I will find one spot of joy in my day."

Courage

Sometimes, showing compassion requires a lot of courage. You might need to step out of your comfort zone and do something unusual.

In his book *Compassion in Practice*, Frank Rogers tells a beautiful story about witnessing an act of compassion at a wedding reception. As people mingled and visited, he noticed an elderly gentleman sitting in a wheelchair toward the edge of the crowd. The man was quiet and didn't speak to anyone.

When the band started to play, many of the guests stood and moved onto the dance floor. After listening to the music for a while, the elderly man rolled his wheelchair to the edge of the dance floor, where he moved and swayed to the music.

A woman at a nearby table had been watching him and followed his movements. Finally, she got up, went over to his wheelchair, bent down and asked him if he wanted to dance. He nodded yes and slowly got up from his chair.

As other couples moved to the side, the two of them danced and when they sat back down, everyone applauded. The man smiled broadly as he thanked her for dancing with him.

Then he added, "It's been 20 years since my wife died and I haven't danced since then. I've missed it so much, partly because when I dance, I feel loved and I feel the power of God lifting me up."

In this case, compassion took courage, but the woman's actions became a rainbow in the elderly man's life.

Remember who you are

As you work on renewing your compassion, take a few moments to look back on your life experiences. Try to remember what you were like during times when you were at your best.

How did you take care of yourself? How did you relate to important people in your life? Were you kind, warm, likeable, approachable? Did you make time for others, even when you were busy?

Remember the days when you felt confident, strong, capable and able to face challenges head-on. Even if it's been years ago, think of times when you were truly at your best in many areas of your life including physically as well as mentally and emotionally.

Our characteristics from the past don't actually leave. But as years go by, we tend to lose sight of our strengths and our gifts. Sometimes we start seeing only the parts of ourselves that we don't like.

To bring back the positive qualities and concepts you've lost, remind yourself that you still value them. Then intentionally put them into your life again.

I suggest you create a list of words and phrases that describe what you are like when you're at your absolute best. As you write your list, think of your best personality traits as well as your skills.

For example, when I am at my best, I am energetic, productive, hard-working and confident about my abilities. I laugh easily, I relate well to people in my life, and I am kind and considerate to others. I regularly read my Bible, pray and cultivate my spirituality. And I make time for those around me and do my best to show compassion to them.

Whenever I look at my list, I'm reminded of how easily I let go of some of those wonderful traits. I let stress or worry or fatigue keep me from showing the best parts of who I am. But since the things on my list describe who I am "at my best," I remind myself that all of these words remain true, even on days when I don't feel or act like them.

Change your routine

Some years ago, one of my students decided it was time to switch things around in his life. After he finished high school, he went to barber school and for eleven years he toiled away at his job as a barber.

But he wasn't happy. He struggled with boring days, doing the same routine over and over, while trying to keep a smile on his face. One day he made a decision to stop being a barber and instead finish college and go to law school. When I met him, he said, "This is a huge jump in my life, but I've gotten back my excitement and compassion for people I want to help."

On the surface, habits are good for us because they provide stability and make life predictable. However, they can also cause us to lose sight of things we value such as caring about others.

Take a look at your own life routines. Are you spending time every day with someone who brings you down? Maybe you need to shake things up and get past the routine that causes that. Your own changes don't need to be as drastic as the ones made by my student. But even small ones can make a significant difference in renewing your passion for life.

One of my friends decided to change the route for her drive home from work, and she discovered a beautiful neighborhood with large trees and parks. Once she got home, she entered her house through the front door instead of through the garage. This gave her a different view of her family members and their needs.

A few weeks after doing these changes, my friend realized she felt renewed and more energetic once she got home. This also gave her more patience to deal with the demands of her home life.

Deeper meaning of compassion

One of my favorite scenes in the movie *The Wizard of Oz* is when Dorothy is walking down a long winding road, arm and arm with the Lion, the Scarecrow and the Tin Man. All four of these characters have faced a lot of challenges, but at this moment, they put those problems aside to travel life's adventures together.

Although she doesn't know it at the time, Dorothy's compassion helps the Lion find his courage, the Scarecrow find his brain, and the Tin Man find his heart. In the beginning of the movie, Dorothy feels lost and afraid, but as she helps her new friends, she finds herself again and rediscovers happiness.

This story demonstrates a deeper meaning of compassion. As we show empathy and caring for others, we discover something wonderful in ourselves. Compassion enables us to be who we truly are inside, someone who cares about the misfortune of others. And by showing compassion, we help those around us not feel so alone.

In my own life, I show compassion because *that is who I am*. I strive to have an identity of being a kind and caring person in this world. My compassion may help others, but it also brings peace and joy to my soul and gives me a sense that my life matters.

CHAPTER 18

Compassion and Happiness

WHEN MY WIFE AND I ARRIVED in a small town in central Nebraska, I felt scared but also excited. I had just finished seminary and was ready to begin my work as a church pastor. Although I had grown up in California and didn't know much about farming or small towns, I was eager to get started.

I especially wanted the church members to like me, and I wanted to get along with the people in my parish. I had a lot of ideas for doing creative things with the worship services, including leading the singing with a guitar. But it didn't take long for me to realize I had a lot to learn.

Within the first few weeks of my new job, I was warned to stay away from a man I will call "old man Brown." He was the oldest of four brothers who lived in the town. They were all staunch church members and well-known in the community.

I was told that "old man Brown" was very traditional, didn't like change, and was powerful enough to make my life miserable. Perhaps I was naïve, but I decided to start by caring about Mr. Brown. So I arranged for an afternoon visit with him at his home.

I began by telling him I didn't know much about rural life, and I would like to hear about his experiences as a farmer over many years. He looked surprised but then began talking about his family and their long history of farming in the area.

For over an hour, I just listened, nodded, and asked a few questions. Then I got up to leave and asked him if I could come back the next week. He said that would be fine, and we shook hands before I left. For the next several weeks, I stopped by for visits and kept asking him more about the challenges of farming.

At the end of one of my visits, I told him I would like to bring my wife along the next time. I asked, "Would it be OK if she brings her guitar and sings for you?" He said that would be fine, and again we shook hands before I left.

When we arrived the next week, Mr. Brown's wife served us tea and homemade cookies. Then my wife played her guitar while quietly singing a couple of well-known hymns. The Browns thanked her and said they loved the music.

At that point, I took a bold step and asked if they would be comfortable with her playing the guitar in church sometime. They both looked a little surprised, but then Mr. Brown said, "That sounded really nice, and I guess it would be fine for her to sing some hymns in church with her guitar."

As time went on, I continued my visits with Mr. Brown. At one point, I asked him to tell me about his experiences at the church. I especially wanted to know where he saw problems and ways he could help me. He said, "I want someone who will listen to us when things don't go well." I assured him that he could count on that. I also visited each of his brothers and their families and asked them to help me as well.

Over the five years I was a pastor at that small church, I never had a problem with the Brown family. We became close friends, and my wife and I were invited to many of their family gatherings. I saw firsthand the outcome of suspending judgments and instead doing actions that help people know someone cares about them. My acts of compassion with this family helped with my work, but it also brought a lot of happiness to my own life.

I am amazed at how showing compassion to others affects me. Even if I'm having a really bad day, doing an act of compassion always makes me feel better. Simply showing caring and concern has an interesting way of improving my mood and making me feel happier.

What is happiness?

In my work, I've often asked people the question, "What defines happiness for you?" I usually hear words such as *contented, satisfied, joyful, cheerful* and *peaceful*. Sometimes, happiness comes when we feel excited about something we're doing or a goal we've achieved. Although the meaning of happiness differs for each of us, the common factor is that we describe it with positive emotions.

Research has been able to demonstrate biological links between acts of compassion and changes in our brain activity. Doing something nice for another person calms our nervous system, slows our heart rate, and stimulates the production of oxytocin, which makes us feel better about ourselves.

These changes affect our facial features by softening our eyes and making our smile more genuine. As a result of our showing compassion, people will perceive us as being warmer and more approachable.

Social psychologist Sonja Lyubomirsky, author of *The How of Happiness*, did an experiment with one of her university classes. To see if compassion affected happiness, she divided her students into two groups. She asked those in one group to do five acts of compassion a week, while those in the second group didn't do any.

The compassionate acts tended to be simple, such as buying a hamburger for a homeless person, putting money in parking meters or visiting someone in the hospital. Other students described buying coffee for strangers or letting someone go ahead of them in a store line.

For six weeks, the students in both groups recorded their emotions. The compassion group described feeling more positive and having a significant increase in their happiness. Dr. Lynbomirsky explains that happiness grows through intentional activities, as opposed to sitting around waiting for something to happen.

In similar research, *The Journal of Happiness Studies* describes an interesting outcome of showing compassion. For six months, research participants agreed to do one small compassionate act every day and then record it in the evening. Nearly all of the participants reported experiencing greater meaning and purpose in their lives, elevating their happiness. But the amazing thing was that their sense of feeling happier continued long after the study ended.

I believe that compassion promotes happiness by derailing the tendency to look at the dark side of life or to be preoccupied with what's wrong. As we show empathy for others, happiness has greater room to grow. In essence, showing compassion helps us look for what's positive in situations and treat people with hope instead of judgment. This helps us view our own life issues with more grace and understanding.

It doesn't take doing great deeds to get the benefit of improved happiness. The types of actions that refocus our brain's circuitry can simply be ones that bring a smile to someone's face.

It might be telling someone, "I was thinking about you today." It may be an expression of gratitude such as, "I am so thankful for you." Or, "I can always count on you." Or it might be a small action such as carrying a heavy box or holding a door for someone.

Compassion changes people

In my university work, I know that professors will often encounter students who can challenge our patience and make teaching difficult. A few years ago, a colleague warned me about a student who would be in my class that was starting the following week.

He told me, "That particular student is a huge problem. She'll constantly interrupt you and she'll dominate class discussions. She won't turn her work in on time and then she'll blame you. I suggest you let her know early on that you won't tolerate any those behaviors."

On the first day of class, I quickly figured out which student he was describing. She had a constant scowl on her face, and she looked distant and unhappy. Since I had a few minutes before class started, I approached this student, welcomed her and asked a few questions about what was important to her.

When the time came for class discussion, I divided the students into groups of twos and fours, which limited anyone from controlling the conversation. Then I asked that student to be part of a group with a few of my best students. She relaxed a little and looked happy about being included.

I also affirmed the student's contributions in the larger class discussions, hoping she didn't feel a need to prove herself. Throughout the semester, I continued to affirm her and offer encouragement about her work. Gradually, she began to appear more comfortable with the other students. She participated well in the class and never showed any of the behaviors I had been warned about.

When the semester ended, this student told me how much the class had meant to her. She said, "I felt the warmth you expressed toward all of us, and it made me feel like I belonged and was accepted." Her feedback meant the world to me, and I realized that showing compassion to her had actually made me extremely happy.

Compassion through good thoughts

To improve your happiness, you might not even have to do an act of compassion. Simply thinking about it can make you feel happier.

In the journal *Emotion*, researchers looked at the effect of visualizing goodwill to others. For seven minutes a day, participants were asked to picture good things happening to others. This included people they didn't get along with and even strangers. They might wish others to have good health, a happier day or success in some endeavor.

The results were fascinating. Compassion expressed through nothing more than warm wishes for people greatly improved the positive moods of the participants. In other words, sending thoughts of goodwill toward others contributes to our own happiness.

When I see someone standing on a street corner while holding a sign that asks for money, I have changed my attitude. I used to sputter to myself, "They look pretty healthy. Why don't they get a job?" Now I try to remember the research on goodwill and send those people warm thoughts for their day and their lives. Sometimes I will say a quick prayer for them as well.

With my new attitude, I don't feel angry or irritated about our social problems in the world. I know I can't solve the issues of homelessness or poverty, but by sending people warm thoughts and a quick prayer, I feel happier about my day.

Surprising ways to promote happiness

Joseph Charles was an unremarkable man by most of the world's standards. He lived in a small home in a quiet neighborhood in Berkeley, California. He was retired from his job and was generally a happy person.

One morning, he decided to share his happiness by waving to the neighbor who lived next door. The man waved back, so Mr. Charles waved to him again the next morning. Then he decided to expand his efforts and he started waving to others from the front of his house.

Eventually, he moved to a nearby street corner and began waving to people as they drove by. For 30 years, Monday through Friday, rain or shine, Mr. Charles stood on that corner, smiling and waving to commuters on their way to work. He even shouted to drivers, "Keep smiling and have a good day."

In the beginning, people thought he was crazy. This included his neighbors, several members of his church, and even his wife. One neighbor decided to call the police, but when the officers arrived, they laughed. They knew they couldn't arrest a man for trying to bring a smile to the hardened faces of people on their way to work.

One day, a driver stopped and gave Mr. Charles a pair of bright yellow gloves. He loved them because they made it easier for people see his arms waving. Over the years, bright yellow gloves became part of his trademark, and drivers would watch for them. Often people would go out of their way to drive past his corner.

Mr. Charles learned that you never know how much your acts of compassion might affect the lives of others. One day a stranger stopped by his home and said, "You don't know me, but my wife and I have been having lots of problems and thought of getting a divorce. But after driving by your house every day and seeing your positive outlook on life, we've decided to give it another try."

The nicest part," said Mr. Charles, "is that a few days later, his wife came by and told me the same thing."

As one of his neighbors walked past him each morning, she often stopped to visit for a few minutes. She said, "He would always give me strength to go on with my day."

When Mr. Charles died, more than two hundred people gathered to remember him and his smiles. The mayor said, "That wonderful man's wave and smile cost no money and required no environmental impact reports or endless meetings. Yet every day, he brought joy to others and improved the quality of life for thousands."

You don't need to begin waving at people on a street corner, but remind yourself that you can be a beacon of happiness to people you encounter in your day. You'll find your own peace and joy growing as a result.

Compassionate relationships are like emotional vitamins that help shorten our negative moods. If you live or work in an environment with a steady diet of negative interactions, you can get worn down. To boost your level of happiness each day, strive to make the number of positive and compassionate interactions outnumber the negative ones.

"Some day"

We all do it at times. We keep thinking that "one of these days," life will change and everything will get better. We find ourselves waiting for the next achievement, the next job change, the next relationship, or the next place to live. But when some things improve, we still have to wait for other things to get better.

Happiness comes when we stop chasing the future and live more in the present. This begins with a healthy dose of self-compassion and slowing down to appreciate the moment. Psychologist Emma Sapporo recommends what she calls "compassionate breathing." She points out that when we feel stressed or anxious, our breath shortens. In fact, this also happens whenever we feel most negative emotions.

We can change this pattern by slowing our breathing and taking deeper breaths. This practice resets the emotions from negative to at least neutral and in some cases, changes them to being more positive.

Lifelong happiness

Every kind act done out of compassion shines a light in the darkness of the world. It creates a few moments of happiness where there may be emptiness or sadness.

A wonderful Chinese proverb says, "If you want happiness for an hour, take a nap. If you want happiness for a year, inherit a fortune. If you want happiness for a lifetime, help someone else."

No act of compassion is too small. You make a difference with each person whose life you touch. Do something kind, then smile. Then do another kindness and smile again.

You have just added to your own happiness.

CHAPTER 19

Compassion Stories

WE MIGHT FORGET many things about our life journeys, but we rarely forget someone's kindness to us during times when we were hurting or in need. These wonderful moments become embedded in our life stories.

When I asked people to share stories of compassion, the response was overwhelming. It seems that most people can recall times when giving or receiving compassion touched their lives.

In this chapter, you will learn from the stories I've heard. Some tell about small but meaningful acts of compassion done by one person. Others relate to times when compassion affected thousands of people. But in every situation, you'll see the power of kindness and the ways it improves our world.

Compassion improved someone's life

Often what seems like a simple act of compassion will leave a lasting benefit for the person who received it. The following stories reflect situations where compassion made a significant difference in someone's life.

Caring at a food pantry

"When I became disabled, I had to leave my job and wasn't able to look for another one. I watched my meager savings slowly disappear until I was down to a couple hundred dollars. That made me eligible for food stamps, so I went to the agency and applied. I felt a little humiliated that I was having to get public assistance, but I really needed the help.

"The person I dealt with at the agency helped me get signed up, then suggested I go across the street to a food pantry. I did. And I'll never forget the kindness of the people at the food pantry as they led me around and explained what and how much I could get. They even piled on extra items. Their compassion for me took away the embarrassment and humiliation I had been feeling.

"That day was years ago, but I'll always remember the kindness of those workers and how much it helped me. I hope I'm always that kind to the people I meet in my own life." *Laura B.*

Learning to read

"A friend's sister was a struggling single mother with two children. One of her daughters was bullied at school because she was overweight, and the distress caused her to have trouble with learning. When the daughter was entering 5th grade, testing showed she didn't know how to read.

"We had a family friend who worked as a tutor, using creative approaches and books that helped kids who had reading problems. I hired this woman, and for one year, I paid for her to tutor my friend's daughter. By the time she entered 6th grade, the daughter was reading at the right level for her age. The girl's mother was so grateful for my help, and I felt happy about doing something that made a difference in someone's life." *June P.*

Kindness of a physician

"When I was diagnosed with heart atrial fibrillation a few years ago, my cardiologist kept encouraging me and telling me things would improve. Each time I ended up in the emergency room, he would stop by and, in a gentle voice, remind me that I would feel better again soon.

"The good news is that medications he prescribed have worked great, and I haven't had any problems for a long time. I've always been amazed at how much those kind words meant to me. They gave me courage and strength at times when I needed them the most." *Linda S.*

A hospital Christmas

"When our father was 85, he developed serious health issues and was hospitalized for several weeks. Because he couldn't go home for Christmas, our family decided to hold our holiday dinner and gift exchange at the hospital. The cafeteria workers moved several tables together and gave us all a free meal.

"Because several family members lived in other states, we arranged to stay overnight at a nearby hotel. That year, the hotel's owners gave free rooms on Christmas Eve and Christmas Day to anyone who had a family member in the hospital. Because most of us were on tight budgets, their generosity was a great help to all of us. We still have warm memories of that Christmas and how compassion made it one of our best holidays." *L.J.*

Return of an angel clip

"Some years ago, my husband and I decided to sell our pickup truck, since we weren't needing it any more. A nice young man named Nick asked to buy the truck, and after we came to a price agreement, he met us at our local bank to complete the sale.

"We had already removed all of our personal items and thoroughly cleaned the truck. So when we handed Nick the keys, we felt happy about the sale. But on the way home, I remembered the 'guardian angel clip' that had been fastened to the passenger's side visor. It was the last thing given to me by my father, and I had kept it to remind us to be safe on the road.

"When I realized I'd forgotten to remove it, I called Nick and asked if he would check to see if the clip was still there. He was already 40 miles away, but he pulled over and told me it was safely attached to the visor. I offered to pay for him to send it to me, but he assured me it was no problem for him to return it.

"The next day, the treasured angel clip arrived in an overnight mail package. Nick's kindness and generosity meant so much to me, especially because of the meaning of that clip and the connection to my dad." *Susan P.*

Encouragement cards

"Instead of sending sympathy cards to people who have lost loved ones, I buy 'encouragement cards.' I especially try to find ones with messages that relate to what a grieving person might be experiencing.

"After studying many cards at a Dollar Tree store, I took quite a few to the checkout counter. But as I watched the clerk ringing them up, I realized she had missed one of the cards. I pointed it out her and assured her I didn't want to cause trouble because of the missed sale. The clerk thanked me profusely for calling it to her attention and said my kindness made a difference in her work and her day." *Sharon L.*

Cancer treatment support

"When I was going through treatment for breast cancer, I struggled with feeling awful related to the medication I had to be on. One day my sister handed me a small, silver medallion inscribed with an angel figure.

"She said a friend had asked her to give it to me and explained, 'I held this medallion a lot during my own cancer treatment and felt the strength from it. Now I am cancer-free and doing great, so it's time for you to have it and draw encouragement and strength from it as well.'

"That was more than twelve years ago, and until recently, I would still pull out that medallion now and then. I knew that some day, I would give it to another person who needed it more than I did, and last month, I was able to do that." *Linda S.*

Compassion among friends

Many times, friends show compassion in small ways that end up meaning a lot to the person who was the recipient. Even a few words in an email or a card can brighten someone's day and bring that person encouragement and support. During painful times such as loss or grieving, a friend's acts of compassion are remembered forever.

Examples from cards and notes

"My dear friend, thank you so much for the sunny flowers you brought me. It is such a comfort to have the care and concern of a good friend." *Thank-you note from Suzanne N.*

"It is believed there are angels on earth. I know there is one watching over me. I can't ever thank you enough for all you did for me while I've been healing from my hip replacement surgery. God has blessed me with you in my life!" *Thank-you note from Marilee F.*

"When I think of 'kindness,' I think of you! Your kind heart has been with me all these months, and I so appreciate it. Just thinking of you brings a smile to my heart." *A card from Barb S.*

"I wanted you to know how grateful I am for you and your work. Your emails always seem to come at the perfect time. I sincerely appreciate all you do and I always look forward to hearing from you. Sending you virtual hugs!" *Email from Felicia F.*

During times of grief and loss

"When a friend's husband died suddenly from a heart attack, a couple of us volunteered to help clean her home. In the bedroom where the man had fallen, we found a blood stain in the carpet. One friend who was a nurse knew how to clean that type of area, and after we worked on it, the stain was completely gone. The grieving friend was so grateful that she didn't have to tackle cleaning that room." *L.J.*

Aaron's last wish

When Aaron Collins passed away just after his 30th birthday, one of his final wishes was to give a waiter or waitress a $500 tip. His brother Seth fulfilled his wish at Puccini's Restaurant in Lexington, Kentucky. He recorded a video of the event, explaining to the waitress, Sarah Ward, that his brother had just passed away and that giving a $500 tip was Seth's final wish.

He posted the video on YouTube, and within days, it had been viewed more than one million times. Since that time, over $30,000 has been donated to continue the cause, now known as "Aaron's Last Wish." For several years, Seth continued to fulfill his brother's wish, and he has given $500 tips to more than a hundred restaurant workers.

Compassion through connecting

Whether it's neighbors, work groups or extended family members, I often hear amazing stories about showing compassion with people you hardly know. After a natural disaster such as a fire, tornado or flood, neighbors or members of a church or community group will often arrive to help clean up the aftermath of the destruction.

In many churches, long-time traditions include serving lunch or coffee and dessert after a funeral. I have often watched the caring spirit of the "mission circle" women as they refilled coffee cups and spoke kind words to grieving family members. Many times, these were people the serving women didn't even know.

Watch for opportunities to show compassion to people who are even distantly connected to you. Pay attention to parents at your child's school, members of your softball league or those in a Sunday School class at your church. Sometimes, you'll learn about someone's need through passing conversations with people in these groups.

Here are stories of people with only a distant connection to those who received their compassion.

Notes from a school principal

At a 2021 high-school graduation in Palm Coast, Florida, on each student's chair was a handwritten note from Jeff Reaves, the school's principal. Over the past three months, Principal Reaves had scoured through transcripts, emails and his own memories in order to mention personal things to each of the 459 graduates.

Students and staff members were equally amazed and appreciative of this unusual way of connecting with all of the graduating seniors. Principal Reaves said, "It was a great experience for me because I got the chance to learn about each student individually. I wanted to help them feel connected and have their high school experiences feel positive."

Farmers and neighbors

"My family runs a dairy farm in a rural community of neighbors who tend to always help each other when needed. One winter, a section of our barn roof collapsed due to the weight of snow. My husband called the fire department, a volunteer group made up mostly of local dairy farmers.

"Several firefighters arrived quickly, and they transported all of our cows to their own farms. For the next two months while our barn was being repaired, these farmers fed our cows and milked them twice a day. In our farming community, this level of kindness happens a lot as we all try to help out our neighbors when needed." *June P.*

When compassion helps lots of people

Most of us don't have opportunities to affect thousands of lives. But by participating in fundraising or donation events, your small contribution can reach people all over the world.

Salvation Army work

When you drop money into the red kettle in December, your donation affects thousands of people. Each year the Salvation Army provides services for more than thirty million people nationwide. This includes feeding, clothing, sheltering and providing disaster relief.

The Salvation Army states that eighty-two cents of each dollar received goes directly toward programming and meeting needs in the communities of the donors.

The amazing sock drive

Each December, Lutheran Church of Hope in Des Moines, Iowa, chooses a specific area of need to focus on during the Advent season. A few years ago, the organizers learned that many individuals coming to the shelters for homeless people had either worn-out socks or no socks at all. So for that year's Advent fundraiser, the church asked for donations of socks.

The socks had to be new, but they could be any size or color. By the end of the sock drive, the church had collected enough pairs of socks to fill thirteen pallet-size Gaylord boxes. This was the equivalent of filling one and a half semi trucks with donated socks.

After serving the local shelters, the leaders spread the sock donations out to shelters in many surrounding towns and rural areas. *Shared by Mike Horstmann, Local Missions Coordinator at Lutheran Church of Hope*

Little Dresses for Africa

A friend named Diana is part of a group of women who make little dresses from pillow cases. The finished garments are sent to Little Dresses for Africa, an international humanitarian group that distributes them to areas where they are needed most.

In the beginning, the little dresses were sent to Africa and given to young girls who otherwise might not have clothes to wear. In recent years, the project has expanded to include sending dresses to many countries hit by disasters, including the United States.

Diana's sewing group meets once a month to work on projects together, but in between, they all make clothing at home for the Little Dresses program. In addition to dresses from pillow cases, many of the sewers make them from cheerful, brightly colored fabric.

Their sewing project now includes using soft knit t-shirts to make shorts for boys, as well as cloth diapers and washcloths. Diana's group has partnered with humanitarian organizations such as Orphan Grain Train and Samaritan's Purse for shipping the clothing to Africa and other underprivileged countries.

Replacing bedding after a house fire

A Shelter House home in Iowa City, Iowa, has served for years as a permanent supportive housing model for those who have experienced homelessness and struggle with mental illness. A couple of years ago, a fire caused major damage, displacing all six tenants and leaving them with only the clothes they were wearing.

Shelter House staff were able to find temporary lodging for the tenants, but the workers also needed to replace most of the household items. Through local news outlets, they requested donations of sheets, blankets, pillows and towels. Within a few hours, they had half of a large garage filled with these items. As people arrived in the parking lot with their donations, many had tears in their eyes as they showed compassion for this vulnerable group of people.

Mini compassion stories

When we asked people for stories about compassion in their lives, we received way more than we could include in this book. Some stories were about ways people showed compassion for others, but we also heard about special ways people received compassion from someone.

We compiled some of these into "mini stories" that we hope will inspire you and give you fresh ideas about the importance of even the simplest acts of compassion.

Here are brief summaries of these stories:

"For a 'Meet your country neighbor' project, my husband and I visited 70 homes within a half mile of our house. The outcome surprised us. In addition to getting to know a lot of neighbors, we learned about ways we could help them in times of need. We babysat, mowed yards, comforted new widows and started a weekly Bible club." *Sharon L.*

"When I've been under a lot of stress, I found that making a pie and giving it away helped me cope. Because older people especially loved my pies, I began taking pieces of pie to some of my elderly neighbors and friends.

"My favorite response was from a 92-year-old man who told me that when he tasted my lemon meringue pie, it was as though he was back in his mother's kitchen. He said that with each bite of my pie, he could feel her love again." *Ann D.*

"When I was going through my divorce and raising four teen-aged kids on my own, I was blessed to receive help and encouragement from many people. It seemed that a hug or smile, hand on my shoulder, supportive words and even financial help always came when I needed it most." *Kate W.*

"During the time when visitors were not allowed at our retirement community, my daughter brought us a special box and left it with the security guard at the front gate. When we opened the box, we found it was filled with snacks, artwork and soap along with Sudoku and coloring books. That creative gift felt like a big, warm hug from our daughter and grandkids." *Ann C.*

The power of stories

When you run out of ideas for ways to show caring to others, ask friends and family members to tell you stories about compassion. In most cases, they can immediately describe wonderful, meaningful times when compassion affected their lives. I encourage you to keep track of your own stories about acts of compassion. First, watch for moments when you can show compassion, then write your experiences in a journal or notebook.

Read your stories often, along with the ones in this book. Even during a really hard time in your life, you will quickly find new ideas for showing compassion. And as you take steps toward caring for others, you'll find healing and comfort in your own life.

CHAPTER 20

Compassion for Life

A FEW YEARS AGO, my wife and I went on a short vacation to Nassau in the Bahamas. After getting a bit lost on a long walk, we requested a taxi to take us back to our hotel. The taxi driver was exceptionally cheerful and positive, even singing as he drove.

Finally, I asked him, "Where do you get so much energy to help others?" He gave me a big smile and thanked me for my question, then began talking.

"It hasn't always been this way," he said. "Six months ago, when the hurricane destroyed much of my home island, I feared for my life. For three days, my wife and I held our children above the constantly rising water in our home.

"By the time we learned a helicopter was coming to rescue us, the water was up to our necks, my children were very ill and one of them was barely conscious. The helicopter pilot hovered above us and the staff helped us climb into a large basket to transport us to a hospital in Nassau. My children all survived and, eventually, we all became healthy again.

"My brother gave us a place to live and helped me get a job as a taxi driver. I was extremely grateful for the kindness and support we received, and now I work to help others. I try to show kindness and compassion to every person who rides in my taxi. It's simply who I am."

My wife and I were shocked at his tragic story and had no idea how to respond. When we reached our hotel, I gave the taxi driver a large tip and said, "I'm so glad you survived, took care of your children and found a way to begin again. I applaud you!"

I realized there were no right words to say. All I could do was respond with compassion and appreciation for this dear man. After he left us at our hotel, we heard him singing again as he drove away.

"It's who I am"

In spite of his painful history, that delightful taxi driver became a compassionate person who plans to stay that way for life. He created an identity that he demonstrates with everyone he meets. Being compassionate for life doesn't mean he won't have hard times or bad days. But he has chosen to show compassion every chance he gets.

We each have different labels or identities that describe our styles and personalities. For example, I am a professor, husband, dog lover and tennis player. But I have also cultivated the label of *compassionate person*. I do my best to live out of that identity every day by being kind toward others, no matter who they are.

In your own life, occasionally remind yourself about *why* you choose to live as a compassionate person. It may be that you like bringing joy into the lives of others. Maybe one of your goals is to help to make the world a better place.

Like our taxi driver, maybe it's how you show gratefulness for those who have cared for you. Perhaps caring for others makes you feel better about yourself. It may be that compassionate living is an extension of God's spirit within you, making you feel called to care for those in need.

Regardless of your personal reasons, keep strengthening your identity of being a compassionate person. Then live each day watching for ways to show this part of yourself.

Compassion changes people

If there ever was a time for a revival of compassion, it is now. Every day, media outlets remind us about the awful things happening in our world. Our familiar response tends to be, "I can't do anything about that."

Except that maybe we *can*.

While we can't fix or even improve those tragedies, we can influence the lives of people in all of the areas where we live and work. Showing compassion makes a difference in every life we touch.

It provides the opportunity to put a smile on someone's face. It brings back optimism where hope has been lost, and it eases the suffering in people's lives. Some days, you may be the only person who speaks kindly to someone who is lonely or sad. Compassion makes a difference.

In the book *A Path with Heart*, Jack Kornfield reminds us, "The things that matter most in our lives are not fantastic or grand. They are the moments when we touch one another, when we are there in the most attentive and caring ways."

Watch for opportunities

Compassion begins in your mind and your heart. It doesn't require money or being part of a large company or an organization. It starts when you notice a need or a struggle, then respond in a helpful manner.

Perhaps you see someone who is emotionally down or having a hard day. You listen without judgment or irritation.

You hug your child or a family member. You thank a colleague for some extra help on your project.

Places to show compassion are all around you, and you don't need to do anything big. Compassionate acts are not measured by size but by the heart that gives them. Sometimes the smallest action can change someone's day and bring joy and happiness.

My wife's mother spent the last years of her life in an assisted living center and a nursing home. Even though her health issues limited her activities, she always tried to show kindness and appreciation to the staff.

One of the ways she did this was to memorize the names of the staff members and call them by name when they entered her room. She even learned how to tell the identical twin brothers apart and call them by their correct names. The care center staff loved her and appreciated her kindness toward them.

Improving empathy

As you know, the three steps for showing compassion are *notice, feel* and *do*. But sometimes we struggle with the second step of feeling empathy. Perhaps we're tired or overwhelmed with life, and we don't feel like caring about others.

We hesitate because we can't imagine what it's like for someone to experience extreme levels of hurt and pain. But to show compassion, we don't have to know what the pain feels like. Instead, we need to recognize it, respect it and respond to it.

Compassion doesn't require saying, "I know how you feel." In fact, sometimes those words make people upset because you aren't experiencing their pain. A recently widowed friend described her reaction when someone told her, "I'm divorced so I know what you're going through." My friend said this comment made her angry because the pain from death of a spouse isn't even close to going through a divorce.

To show your empathy for someone, use words such as, "I can see that you're hurting. How can I help?" Sometimes it's enough to acknowledge the pain or stress of someone's situation. To do this, you might use the phrase, "My heart is with you."

You may not even get a reply to your words. But often people will respond by saying, "Just knowing that you care helps me."

Even the smallest acts of compassion can be remembered for a long time. One of my students contacted me 15 years after she graduated from college. She described being grateful for the encouragement I gave her to make some changes in her life. She said, "You were there at the right time for me. Your help and input made a wonderful difference in my life."

Outcomes of compassion

After School Matters is a nonprofit organization that provides after-school and summer opportunities for high school teens in the city of Chicago. The brainchild of two strong women, Maggie Daley and Lois Weisberg, this organization initially recruited and paid professional Chicago artists for a unique after-school program.

In addition to helping the teens learn about art, the instructors emphasize the importance of showing up every day, on time and ready to work. The student participants receive a small monetary stipend along with the chance to discover their creativity and express themselves through art.

Since 1991, After School Matters has served more than 350,000 Chicago teens. It's also known as the nation's largest and most successful provider of after-school and summer programs for high school students. It now offers project-based programs in the arts, communications and leadership, sports and STEM (science, technology, engineering and mathematics.) After School Matters has received generous financial support from well-known celebrities as well as the city of Chicago. These donations have helped the program grow and provide buildings for the meetings and training.

But the program participants describe the empathy and compassion of the leaders as having made all the difference in their lives. In many cases, the teens believe the program protected them from the influence of gangs and crime.

Every time you show people compassion, you have the potential to change the outcome of their lives. This is true whether you volunteer, donate money or actually do an act of compassion.

Showing compassion not only helps others but also influences them to take similar actions. For example, children tend to mimic what they see done by their parents. In organizations and neighborhoods, people tend to adopt the behaviors done by others.

Compassion for difficult people

Most of us know a few difficult people who are hard to care about. Our natural tendency is to avoid these people so we don't have to deal with them. In some cases, for our own emotional well-being, that may be the best course of action.

But for many people, compassionate action is a good investment, especially if it's a family member. Sometimes it helps to learn more about what caused a person to become unhappy or angry. Other times, we have to focus on making allowances for people's faults.

Pastor Mike Housholder serves as the senior pastor for Lutheran Church of Hope, a multi-site mega church in Des Moines, Iowa. Between worshipping online and in-person, tens of thousands of people take part in Hope's weekly services. This church demonstrates compassion in dozens of ways through ministries including Celebrate Recovery, Alcoholics Anonymous meetings and significant donations to food banks and world missions. While Rev. Housholder is an outstanding preacher and businessman, he consistently greets parishioners and stays in touch with those facing challenges.

A few months ago, his sermon focused on ways to reach out and care about others, even those who are especially challenging. He said, "Sometimes it helps to label certain people as EGR. That stands for *extra grace required* to love them. Once you understand that, you'll find it easier to show compassion to even the most difficult ones."

Sometimes, you can come up with sneaky ways to show compassion to difficult people. For example, you can wear them down with acts of kindness. Routinely showing them compassion may keep the door open for positive change.

Intentional compassion may require showing extra patience and deflecting problematic comments. Not reacting to difficult people takes away their power. When people verbally attack you, go "emotionally deaf" to their negative talk. Don't take everything personally or assume they are determined to harm you.

Realize their behavior is probably not about you. Most of the time there's something else going on in their lives. So instead of getting angry, mentally reframe their statements to make them sound less challenging. If someone snaps at you about a minor incident, tell yourself, "What that person really meant to say was...," then finish the sentence differently.

You can actually have fun with this by "hearing" the words you would have preferred. For example, when my friend Kimberly returned from lunch and her boss growled, "Where have you been?" she responded by saying, "Hi, did you miss me?"

Compassion requires wisdom

When you are unsure about what to do around difficult people, remember that compassion must be connected to wisdom. Ask yourself, "What is the best way to help this person?" In some cases, the answer may be, "Do nothing."

Other times, you might direct your compassion to groups that can provide the help that is needed. This might include food banks, homeless shelters and other community services. Churches and public agencies can often provide help that is well beyond what we could do by ourselves.

Lead with your heart

In your efforts to be compassionate for life, look for ways to lead with your heart. Most people need grace as much as you do. Others want a second chance and an opportunity to repair their lives. For people feeling alone and forgotten, you may be the only person with enough courage to welcome them back into a community.

Action for Happiness is an international movement with hundreds of thousands of members committed to building a happier and more caring society. They focus on big questions such as, "What really matters in our lives? What really makes us happy?"

They encourage their members to live with the pledge, "I will try to create more happiness and less unhappiness in the world around me."

The organization recommends living by principles of compassion that contribute to happiness. Here are ways for doing this:

- Look for the good in those around you.
- Find three good things in each day.
- Ask others about what is going well for them.
- Do kind things for others.
- Help a friend in need.
- Thank the people you're grateful for.

Keep the steps to compassion foremost in your life. Notice people and situations around you. Build a sense of empathy and caring for them. Take actions that will help relieve suffering and demonstrate caring. In other words:

See, Feel, and Do.

One person can make all the difference in the world, and there's every reason for that person to be _you_.

I AM CLOSING THIS BOOK with a prayer attributed to Saint Francis of Assisi. His words provide a model for all of us to live compassionately in our lives.

Lord, make me an instrument of Your peace.
Where there is hatred, let me sow love;
Where there is injury, pardon;
Where there is doubt, faith;
Where there is despair, hope;
Where there is darkness, light;
Where there is sadness, joy.

O Divine Master,
Grant that I may not so much seek
To be consoled as to console;
To be understood as to understand;
To be loved as to love.

For it is in giving that we receive;
It is in pardoning that we are pardoned;
And it is in dying that we are born to eternal life.

Resources and Websites

Reflections

IN THIS SECTION, you will find examples of quiet reflections which are designed to help you focus and redirect your thoughts. You can use them to calm your stress as well as to nurture positive thoughts and mental images. These are especially helpful during times when you are struggling to show caring and compassion.

The reflections can be used as a "quieting time" or, if you are comfortable with it, as a prayer time to nurture your compassion. When your spirit is quiet and you feel centered and peaceful, you are more able to be patient, forgiving and compassionate toward others.

Instructions

While each of the reflections has a slightly different goal, you can use the same steps to prepare for the experience.

Prepare for doing a reflection by sitting in a quiet place where you feel comfortable and safe and you will not be distracted. Sit in a manner that relaxes your body. Take several slow, deep breaths and let go of any busy thoughts or images.

Relax your shoulders and let go of the stress of the day. Depending on what's most comfortable, you can do these reflections with your eyes open or closed.

During the reflections, you might notice that your mind will tend to wander. That's fine, and it happens to everyone. When it does, simply take note of it and bring your attention back to the exercise. To re-focus, pay attention to your breath and the sensation of breathing in and breathing out.

While it's helpful to do these reflections in order, it isn't necessary. When you are ready to sit quietly and focus, choose the one that fits your needs best at that time. Each of the reflections can be completed in about ten minutes.

As you read the words for each reflection, you can mentally review them or even whisper or pray each of the statements. There's no right or wrong way to use these tools. They simply provide an easy yet structured way to focus your attention and strengthen your ability to show compassion.

Here are the four reflections:

Reflection 1: Self-care
Reflection 2: Just like me
Reflection 3: Loving kindness
Reflection 4: Do it anyway

Reflection 1: SELF-CARE

On days when you feel especially burdened and tired, use this reflection to re-center yourself and remember your inner strength. Ten minutes of focused attention can help you draw on the personal skills and resources you already have. By renewing your belief in yourself, you will rediscover your ability to show kindness and caring toward others.

Review the general instructions, then, once you are seated comfortably, focus your attention on your breathing. Invite good air into your lungs and let go of the bad air. Let your back, your shoulders and your legs go soft and limber.

Center your thinking on each of the following phrases one at a time. Feel free to add additional phrases that have meaning for you.

- I am safe.
- I release my stress into the air.
- As I relax, I am getting stronger.
- I let go of anxiety and I feel peace.
- I am strong and capable.
- I am loved and appreciated.
- God is with me and His angels protect me.

If you notice that your attention has wandered, simply bring it back to the last phrase you chose.

Some people find it helpful to develop their own phrases, and use ones that comfort and draw on inner strength.

Reflection 2: JUST LIKE ME

This reflection involves two parts. The first section reminds you that in many ways, people you care about are just like you. The second part helps you explore ways that a challenging or unhappy person is also just like you.

With each part of this exercise, let yourself feel what it's like to be the person you are picturing as you say or think the phrases of the reflection.

Between the two parts of the reflection, allow yourself 30 seconds of silence. Take several slow, deep breaths before you begin the next section.

1. Someone easy to care for

For this reflection, focus on a good friend, a child, or your spouse or partner. Choose a person who is easy to care for.

If you like, you can imagine this person is sitting next to you or in front of you. Once you have this person clearly in your mind, say or think each of these phrases:

- This person has feelings, emotions and thoughts, just like me.
- This person has at some point been sad, disappointed or angry, just like me.
- This person has experienced physical pain, just like me.
- This person has experienced emotional pain, just like me.
- This person wishes to be free from pain and suffering, just like me.
- This person wishes to be safe, healthy and loved, just like me.
- This person wishes to be happy, just like me.

Close this part of the reflection by sending positive thoughts and wishes toward the person you've been focusing on. Say or think these phrases:

I wish for this person to have strength, resources and social support to navigate the difficulties in life. I wish for this person to be free from pain and suffering.

I wish this because this person is a human being, just like me.

Take a 30-second break here. Focus on doing some slow, deep breathing.

2. Someone difficult or challenging to care for

Now, think about someone who has been challenging for you to get along with. Perhaps this will be someone you've had a difficult time accepting. It might even be someone from your past who still brings you sadness, anger or other negative emotions.

If you like, you can imagine this person is sitting next to you or in front of you. Once you have this person clearly in your mind, say or think each of these phrases:

- This person has feelings, emotions and thoughts, just like me.
- This person has at some point been sad, disappointed or angry, just like me.
- This person has experienced physical pain, just like me.
- This person has experienced emotional pain, just like me.
- This person wishes to be free from pain and suffering, just like me.

- This person wishes to be safe, healthy and loved, just like me.
- This person wishes to be happy, just like me.

Close this part of the reflection by sending positive thoughts and wishes toward the person you've been focusing on. Say or think these phrases:

I wish for this person to have the strength, resources and social support to navigate the difficulties in life. I wish for this person to be free from pain and suffering.

I wish this because this person is a human being, just like me.

As you finish this reflection, spend a few minutes thinking about what you have in common with others. Consider your wishes and dreams for your life. Then review how they compare with the wishes and dreams of the people you chose for this exercise.

Close your reflection by considering ways you could show kindness and caring to one of these people if given the chance.

Reflection 3: LOVING KINDNESS

Begin by sitting in a place where you feel relaxed and safe as well as where you know there won't be a lot of distractions. Ideally, choose a public place where there are other people around. You might consider going to a park or sitting outside a store at a mall. Make sure you choose a place where you will feel comfortable to sit for about ten minutes.

Breathe gently throughout this reflection. Relax your shoulders and let go the stress of the day. Depending on what's comfortable, you may close your eyes or keep them open.

Anytime you begin to feel distracted or forget what you are focusing on, bring your attention back to your breath and the sensation of breathing in and breathing out.

This reflection has four parts. For each part you will mentally focus on one specific individual. Allow 30 seconds of silence after each part.

1. Pick a good friend

Choose someone you find very easy to love. Picture looking at that person in a way that communicates kindness. Then think, whisper or pray goodwill toward this person with the following phrases:

- *May you be safe from danger.*
- *May you be well in body and mind.*
- *May you be free from suffering.*
- *May you be at peace and happy.*

Allow for a 30-second break.

2. Pick a stranger

If you are in a public place, choose a person walking past or sitting nearby. If there is no one around, you can bring to mind someone you might see occasionally at school or work. You can also think of someone you know, but not very well.

In your mind, picture this person sitting next to you or in front of you. Then think, whisper or pray goodwill toward this person with the following phrases:

- *May you be safe from danger.*
- *May you be well in body and mind.*
- *May you be free from suffering.*
- *May you be at peace and happy.*

Allow for a 30-second break.

3. Pick someone challenging for you

This may be a person who irritates you, disappoints you, frustrates you or makes you angry. Picture this individual right in front of you or next to you. Once again, think, whisper or pray goodwill toward this person with the following phrases:

- *May you be safe from danger.*
- *May you be well in body and mind.*
- *May you be free from suffering.*
- *May you be at peace and happy.*

Allow for a 30-second break.

4. Picture all three of them

Now imagine all three of these people together... the good friend who is easy to love, the stranger or acquaintance you don't know very well, and the challenging person who frustrates you. Picture all of you sitting together around a table or in a quiet room.

Think, whisper or pray each of these phrases, wishing goodwill toward everyone in the group:

- *May you be safe from danger.*
- *May you be well in body and mind.*
- *May you be free from suffering.*
- *May you be at peace and happy.*

Close your reflection by considering ways you could show kindness and caring to any one of these people if given the chance.

Reflection 4: DO IT ANYWAY

In this reflection, you will practice the skill of accepting life's disappointing moments, but remaining strong in spite of them.

In the book *Do It Anyway*, Dr. Kent M. Keith describes what he calls "The Paradoxical Commandments." Rather than being upset or frustrated by people's actions, he suggests being kind and positive in spite of the situation.

The goal of this reflection is to help us find personal meaning in the face of adversity and focus on the power we have, rather than lamenting about how helpless we are.

Once again, find a quiet and relaxing space. Allow yourself to accept that life has disappointing moments, gaps between where you are and want to be, and people who may let you down.

As you think about your life, think, whisper or pray these phrases and allow them to give you strength.

- People will disappoint me and sometimes not treat me well; forgive them anyway.
- If I am kind, people may take advantage of my generosity; be kind anyway.
- If I am successful, I might displease those who are jealous; succeed anyway.
- If I am honest and frank, people may disagree with me; be honest and frank anyway.
- If I spend years building something, people might be critical; build it anyway.
- If I find serenity and happiness, others may be jealous; be happy anyway.
- The good I do today, people will often forget tomorrow; do good anyway.

- I will give the world the best I have, knowing it may never be enough; give my best anyway.

As you strive to be a caring, compassionate person, remember that even the smallest kindness matters and can change a person's life forever.

Helpful Links

THIS SECTION INCLUDES website listings for programs and resources mentioned in *Acts of Compassion*.

International Charter for Compassion
https://charterforcompassion.org/charter

Family caregiver alliance
www.caregiver.org

Little Dresses for Africa
https://littledressesforafrica.org

After School Matters
www.afterschoolmatters.org

Action for Happiness International
https://actionforhappiness.org

Acts of Compassion
www.CompassionateForLife.com

Acts of Compassion
Discussion Guides

Available for free download

For participants

This *Acts of Compassion* discussion guide provides a helpful resource for church programs, small groups and book clubs. The guide will help prompt conversations and insights as group members explore the challenges of showing compassion to others as well as to themselves.

Designed for eight sessions, the guide can also be used for longer classes and group meetings as well as individual study. Each session includes excerpts from *Acts of Compassion*, related scriptures and thought-provoking discussion questions.

For leaders

This separate guide for teachers and group leaders includes conversation starter questions along with brief instructions for effectively leading an *Acts of Compassion* discussion group.

To download these free guides, go to:

www.CompassionateForLife.com

Notes

Introduction
https://www.facebook.com/mistystarr.whittingtonrobertson.
Permission granted to be included in this book.

Chapter 1 How It Begins
Research by Emma Seppala and Cendri Hutcherson, 2008, at
California Institute of Technology, https://tinyurl.com/7-
minutes
Leo Buscaglia, https://tinyurl.com/Leo-Buscaglia.
Louis Cozolino, *The Neuroscience of Human Relationships* (New
York: WW Norton, 2006), pp. 13–14.

Chapter 2 How Compassion Works
Brené Brown, *Dare to Lead* (New York: Random House, 2019), p. 142.

Chapter 4 Compassion Heals and Connects
Emotion journal study on relationships, https://tinyurl.com/
Emotion-Journal

Chapter 5 Compassion Helps Both People
Clifton Parker, "Stanford research: It helps well-being," https://
tinyurl.com/helps-well-being
United Health Care mission, statement, https://tinyurl.com/United-
Health-Care
"Can 40 seconds of compassion reduce patient anxiety?" by
L. Fogarty, B. Curbow, and M. Somerfield, *Journal of Clinical
Oncology*, 1999.
Scott Pious' course has enrolled 750,000 students since 2013.
https://www.socialpsychology.org/teach/compassion.htm

Chapter 7 Compassion and the Brain

Andrew Dreitcer, *Living Compassion* (Nashville: Upper Room, 2017), pp. 101–102.

Chapter 8 Self-compassion

Tara Cousineau, *The Kindness Cure* (Oakland, CA: New Harbinger, 2018).

Brené Brown, https://tinyurl.com/Brene-Brown

Brené Brown, *The Gifts of Imperfection* (New York: Random House, 2010), p. 61.

Roy Bennett, *The Light in the Heart* (Roy Bennett, 2016), p. 8.

Chapter 9 Receiving Compassion

Rick Hansen, *Hardwiring Happiness* (New York: Harmony, 2013).

Fred Bryant and Joseph Veroff, *Savoring* (Mahwah, New Jersey: Lawrence Erlbaum, 2007).

Robert Emmons, https://tinyurl.com/Robert-Emmons

Chapter 10 Compassion in Communities

Henri Nouwen, Donald McNeill and Douglas Morrison, *Compassion* (New York: Image Books, 1983).

Dola Dolls bring joy, calm, to dementia patients, https://tinyurl.com/Dola-Dolls, *The Courier*, Findlay, Ohio, April 7, 2021.

The woman who made the wave happen, KCRG News, September 22, 2017, https://tinyurl.com/The-UI-Wave

Chapter 11 Compassion in Organizations

Jonathan Reckford, *Our Better Angels* (New York: St Matthew's Essentials, 2019).

International Charter for Compassion, https://charterforcompassion.org/charter

Chapter 12 Compassion in Churches

Olivia Graham, Diocese of Oxford | Compassionate (anglican.org)

Chapter 13 Compassion and Work

"Hy-Vee cashier helped customer who was short $12, and his kindness is being rewarded in big way," https://tinyurl.com/Hy-Vee-customer, *The Gazette*, Cedar Rapids, Iowa, February 8, 2021.

John Chambers, "Former Cisco CEO John Chambers is trying to change the world," December 3, 2018, https://tinyurl.com/Cisco-John-Chambers

Patagonia and its culture, Bruce M. Anderson, September 27, 2019, https://tinyurl.com/Patagonia-Culture

Jane Dutton, et al." Leading in times of trauma," *Harvard Business Review*, 2002 (January), 54–62.

Kindness study at Coca Cola, "Everyday prosociality in the workplace: The reinforcing benefits of giving, getting, and glimpsing," J. Chancellor et al., *Emotion*, 2018, 507–517.

Scott Kriens, "Compassion & Business?" https://tinyurl.com/Compassion-Business

Jimmy Carter, "God and the presidency: Jimmy Carter on the demands of faith," October 14, 2016, Joseph Hartropp, https://tinyurl.com/Jimmy-Carter-Faith

Chapter 14 Compassion and Forgiveness

Everett Worthington, *Forgiving and Reconciling* (Downers Grove, Illinois), p. 42.

Maya Angelou, *Letter to My Daughter* (New York: Random House, 2008), p. xii.

Chapter 15 Barriers to Compassion

Paul Gilbert, "Explorations into the nature and function of compassion," *Current Opinion in Psychology*, 2019, 28:108–114.

Peter Singer, *The Most Good that You Can Do* (New Haven: Yale University Press, 2015).

Chapter 16 Compassion Fatigue
Paul Gilbert, "How to turn your brain from anger to compassion,"
https://tinyurl.com/Anger-to-compassion
Family caregiver alliance, https://www.caregiver.org

Chapter 17 Compassion Renewal
Frank Rogers, *Compassion in Practice* (Nashville: Upper Room
Books, 2016).

Chapter 18 Compassion and Happiness
Sonja Lyubomirsky interview by Caitland Fairchild, January 13,
2020, https://tinyurl.com/The-Renewal-Project
Myriam Mongrain, Jacqueline M. Chin and Leah B. Shapira, *Journal
of Happiness Studies*, 2011, 963–981.
Cendri A. Hutcherson, Emma M. Seppala, and James J. Gross,
Loving-Kindness Meditation Increases Social Connectedness,
Emotion, 2008, 720–724.
Joseph Charles, https://berkeleycitizen.org/memoriam/
memoriam12.htm

Chapter 19 Compassion Stories
Little Dresses for Africa, https://littledressesforafrica.org/.
Jeff Reaves, principal of Matonzas High School, Palm Coast,
Florida, *Daytona Beach News-Journal*, June 6, 2021.

Chapter 20 Compassion for Life
Jack Kornfield, *A Path with a Heart* (New York: Bantam, 1993) p. 14.
After School Matters, https://www.afterschoolmatters.org
Action for Happiness International, https://actionforhappiness.org

About the Authors

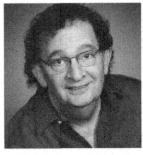

MICHAEL SPANGLE, PhD, has been a communications professor at Regis University in Denver, Colorado. For the past 25 years he has taught courses in forgiveness, emotions, persuasion, conflict management, negotiation and mediation.

As a professional mediator, he has helped organizations and individuals find solutions to conflict and settle long-standing disputes. In the Denver area, he has provided mediation for industries, city governments, schools, churches and hospitals.

Prior to working in higher education, Dr. Spangle served 16 years as a Chaplain in the U.S. Navy Reserve and 15 years as a church pastor. In addition to his doctorate degree, he also holds masters degrees in counseling, ministry and education.

Dr. Spangle has co-authored four books as well as published many journal articles in his fields of study. His book, *Forgiving Others, Forgiving Ourselves*, has been used as a learning guide for churches and small groups.

For information on Mike's books and mediation work as well as contact information, visit: **www.CompassionateForLife.com**

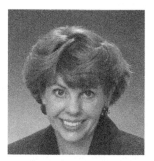

LINDA SPANGLE, RN, MA, has been recognized nationally as a leading authority on emotional eating and other psychological issues of weight management.

A registered nurse with a master's degree in health education, Linda is a skilled teacher, counselor and writer. She is the owner of Weight Loss for Life, a healthy lifestyles coaching and training program.

Linda is the author of five internationally acclaimed books that address weight-loss barriers such as emotional eating, low motivation and sabotage. Several of her books, including *Life Is Hard, Food Is Easy* and *Friends with the Scale*, have won national awards.

In addition to being interviewed by hundreds of radio shows, newspapers and magazines, Linda has been a guest on numerous TV shows including Fox News and Lifetime TV. She has been quoted in nearly every major women's magazine, including *Shape*, *Women's Day* and *O Magazine*.

For information on Linda's books and coaching programs as well as contact information, visit: **www.WeightLossJoy.com**

For *Acts of Compassion* resources and free
discussion guides for churches and small groups, visit:

www.CompassionateForLife.com

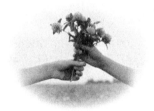